STOLEN MIND

STOLEN MIND

THE SLOW DISAPPEARANCE
OF RAY DOERNBERG

by Myrna Doernberg

With an introduction by
Barry W. Rovner, M.D.

Algonquin Books of Chapel Hill
1986

Algonquin Books of Chapel Hill
Post Office Box 2225
Chapel Hill, N.C. 27515–2225

© 1986 by Myrna Doernberg. All rights reserved.
Introduction © 1986 by Barry W. Rovner
Printed in the United States of America

To Michael and David, who are a tribute to
their dad.

To my parents, Ida and Charles Lazarov,
and my sister Deena Strome for
their love and support.

For Ray, whom I loved deeply and completely.

The water is wide, I cannot cross o'er.
And neither have I the wings to fly.
Give me a boat that can carry two,
And both shall row, my love and I.

Thanks . . .
to all the friends who listened and gave me
strength.

Special thanks to Dr. Frank Wood, Dr. Maureen
Elliott, Rudolph Sommer, Jan Marion, Harolene
Tucker, and John Shaffner for their encouragement
and help.

My sincerest appreciation to Garrett Epps, a
sensitive and sincere editor, for his guidance and
understanding.

INTRODUCTION

Barry W. Rovner, M.D.

Dementia Research Clinic, The Johns Hopkins Hospital,
Baltimore, Maryland

This is the story of a bright and vigorous man in his forties who progressively loses his memories and his understanding of his world, of himself, and of the lives of the people he loves.

His wife begins to write this account as she cares for him and witnesses the change. She—like many now, and as more will do in the future—provides care for someone who is gradually but inexorably slipping away, not physically but mentally. This is a story about a man with a rare and untreatable neurological disease, but it is also a story about families, about love, and ultimately about what it means to be human.

Understanding how individuals think, feel, and act necessarily draws us to a study of the brain. Yet all individuals experience thinking, feeling, and acting not in their brains, but in that realm of personal consciousness called "mind." The relationship of brain and mind is a mysterious one, for "suddenly the phenomena we describe change from tangibles such as cells, neurons, or brains to intangibles such as thoughts, moods, or intentions" (P. R. McHugh and P. R. Slavney, *The Perspectives of Psychiatry* [Baltimore, Md., 1983]). Both the perspective of brain and the perspective of mind are needed to comprehend human lives, but it is almost impossible to use those two perspectives simultaneously.

As we read Myrna Doernberg's account, for example, we see her husband Ray in two very different ways—first as a person or subject troubled in understandable ways, then as an organism or object crippled by a diseased brain. For Myrna Doernberg, the parallax is dizzying. The borderland between mind and brain, between person and organism, becomes a quagmire in which she struggles to comprehend the progressive mental deterioration of her husband. Caught between a "psychological" perspective (Ray willfully dependent) and a "biological" perspective (Ray impaired by disease), she is buffeted by uncertainty and frustration. Not knowing is bad enough, but even worse for Mrs. Doernberg is the day-to-day fact of her husband's existence. He is at once familiar and profoundly changed, at once there and absent.

In retrospect, it is clear that the changes in Ray's thoughts, moods, and acts arose fundamentally from damage to his brain. Ray suffered from subcortical arteriosclerotic encephalopathy or Binswanger's disease, a progressive degeneration of the subcortical regions of the brain caused by severe narrowing of blood vessels and small strokes. The nerve cells of the subcortex allow us to move voluntarily, to perceive our environment, and to maintain attention and consciousness. "Thinking," per se, may be said to occur in the overlying cortex, but the ability to think normally depends on the integrity of the subcortex. Disruption in the subcortex produces profound changes in the organized course of all mental activity.

Clinically, Binswanger's disease appears as a dementia syndrome, a deterioration of intellectual capacity characterized by disturbances in memory, orientation, language, and performance of tasks, with loss of initiative and emotional responsiveness, low frustration tolerance, poor judgment, and an eventual loss of awareness that such changes are occurring. Such difficulties are never part of normal aging, and always represent a disease process.

There are many diseases that cause dementia besides Binswanger's disease. In fact, Binswanger's disease is quite rare. When Otto Binswanger originally described the disease in 1894, he reported on eight patients with progressive dementia syndromes associated with subcortical degeneration. Around that time, physicians were beginning to differentiate dementing illnesses from one another by examination of the brain at autopsy. So, for example, in 1907 Alois Alzheimer described the cortical degeneration characteristic of the disease that bears his name. Alzheimer's disease and Binswanger's disease resemble each other clinically in many ways; however, approximately a million people suffer from Alzheimer's disease while fewer than one hundred cases of Binswanger's disease have been reported. The three most frequently encountered dementing conditions are Alzheimer's disease, multi-infarct dementia, and normal pressure hydrocephalus. The psychological and behavioral changes in a given demented individual are determined by the underlying disease illness. Thus, the effects of dementia will differ from time to time in a given person and even differ to a certain extent from one demented patient to another. While many of the psychological and behavioral changes described above are features of both Alzheimer's disease and Binswanger's disease, there are important distinctions. Alzheimer's disease affects predominantly the cortex of the brain and has characteristic pathological changes: tangles of protein fibers (neurofibrillary tangles) and accumulations of degenerating nerve cells (neuritic plaques in the brain). In contrast, Binswanger's disease is associated with hypertension and small strokes, leading not only to psychological and behavioral changes, but also to neurological symptoms such as weakness of the limbs, numbness, and epileptic seizures.

Multi-infarct dementia (MID), like Binswanger's disease, is caused by disease of the blood vessels. In MID, however, the multiple infarcts, or strokes, are usually due to small clots originating from the heart or from blood vessels outside the brain. The strokes are only infrequently due to disease of the small blood vessels within the brain itself, and rarely, if ever, are confined to the subcortex, as in Binswanger's disease.

Normal pressure hydrocephalus (NPH) is a potentially reversible dementing condition, which Ray Doernberg's doctors initially suspected was the cause of his difficulties. NPH is characterized by an excess of the cerebrospinal fluid that normally circulates in and around the brain. When there is too much fluid present, the reservoirs (ventricles) containing it enlarge, and the brain is compressed. In addition to dementia,

NPH also produces difficulty in walking and urinary incontinence. (This distinguishes it clinically from Binswanger's disease.) Draining cerebrospinal fluid from the ventricles into the
abdomen may produce dramatic improvement. In Binswanger's
disease the ventricles are also enlarged, not because there is too
much cerebrospinal fluid, but because the brain tissue surrounding them has shrunk. It is for that reason that the shunt
procedure offered no benefit for Ray.

While most dementias are irreversible, treatable medical
conditions such as hypothyroidism and pernicious anemia may
appear as dementia syndromes; they are reversible. Patients
who show signs of dementia should be checked for endocrine
problems or nutritional deficiencies; proper treatment may
cure their mental problems. Furthermore, cognitive change can
be a symptom of certain psychiatric disorders such as depression and delirium. Because both occur in the elderly, they are
often misidentified as irreversible dementias. In fact, recognizing an abnormal mood state (depression) or an alteration in
consciousness (delirium) can lead to appropriate treatment and
an end to the mental problems.

The precise cause of Binswanger's disease is unknown; but a
number of hypotheses have been proposed. The narrowing and
occlusion of small blood vessels in the subcortex reduce the
supply of oxygen and essential nutrients to the area. This may
lead to damage in the brain similar to what occurs in the heart
as a result of high blood pressure and atherosclerosis. The degeneration of the subcortex may also be due to excessive leak-
age of fluid from damaged blood vessels leading to local metabolic imbalance and insufficient oxygen.

Though its cause is unknown, it is clear that Binswanger's
disease is exceedingly rare and that it shares so many clinical
features with other dementia syndromes that physicians cannot diagnose it with certainty. The diagnosis must be confirmed at autopsy. Seen in retrospect, the nature and course of
Ray's deterioration are characteristic of Binswanger's disease.
Early on, however, doctors interpreted his difficulties as signs
of a purely psychological disorder and recommended psycho-

therapy. Had he been assessed by someone trained to recognize neurological and psychiatric disorders, the proper clinical diagnosis—a dementia syndrome—might have been made much earlier. In the end, the signs of a degenerative brain disease—slurred speech, numbness, weakness, and the relentless loss of memory, motor skills, and insight—were all too evident.

Speaking in terms of diseases is not, however, speaking in terms of individuals—it is not speaking in terms of Ray and Myrna Doernberg and their life together. Ray's apparent detachment and loss of insight are the most merciful aspects of the disease; for his wife, they are the source of greatest pain. The "loss" of Ray while he is still physically present generates much of the anger and fear, guilt and blame and—ultimately—the sadness she experiences. Her uncertainty takes the form of torturing and unanswerable questions that recur throughout the story like the symptoms of the disease itself: What does he know? What can he do? Does he still love me? She writes:

> Sometimes I feel like I have a big hole in my stomach. It's open, and empty, and so painful. It aches and begs to be filled, with a touch, some sign of understanding, something that will somehow bond Ray and me again. I don't know how to make the pain go away. But he isn't here for me. He doesn't know that I hurt and can't make the emptiness and loneliness go away. And, yet, he is physically there.
>
> Desperately and continuously I attempt to stir what was. But there is an impenetrable mesh screen that keeps us from touching one another. He stands before me. He looks like the Ray I know. But he is different. Unsuccessful, frustrating, and terrifying as it is, I continue to try to reach through the mesh hoping to reach one small piece of him.

Caught between her urge to escape and her urge to share her husband's destiny, Myrna Doernberg becomes a witness. She finds purpose and meaning in her record and offers it to us. But, she is not alone in this tragedy. As the population ages and more people are at risk to develop dementing conditions, dementia will become part of the lives of thousands of individuals and their families. Dementia is now recognized to be a major health problem, afflicting approximately 10 percent of Americans over sixty-five. At least half of demented individuals have

Alzheimer's disease. Most of them are cared for in their homes, usually by family members, because family care is desired by a majority of Americans. Such caregiving, however, can be stressful; those who give it may find that their own health suffers as a result. There has been all too little concern for patients and their families, and it is therefore understandable why Alzheimer's disease and other dementias have been called "the silent epidemic."

One reason that the devastation produced by dementia syndromes is not more fully appreciated is that its victims have no voice. They seem not to be suffering or even to be dying, just dissolving, missing. We witness ghostly transformations: people who were loving and loved become morbid distortions of themselves. What is gone is personhood—the characteristic thoughts, feelings, and actions that make a human being a person. The cruelest twist is that family and friends see and hear the victim each day in ways reminiscent of how he or she was before. It is a peculiar dissolution of mental life that leaves intact the human form and takes what is most human from it. Furthermore, in contrast to many diseases that we see as afflictions of an individual, this disease includes family members among its victims. Alzheimer's disease has been said to rob the mind of the victim and the hearts of the victim's family. We speak of the mind as stolen, of life denied—as if the result of a criminal act for which there is no recourse, no recompense, no recovery. There is nothing to blame, nothing to see. In this disease, the outcome, death, is not as horrible as the "absence" of the victim in life.

Myrna Doernberg touches on a widespread perception of nursing homes as undesirable. In fact, 20 percent of persons over age sixty-five will reside in a nursing home during their lives. Improving care for elderly patients in nursing homes will become increasingly important as the population ages and more persons require nursing home care. Recognizing potentially reversible mental disorders and initiating appropriate treatment are imperative. Appropriate psychiatric care in nursing homes will require expert psychiatric consultation to encourage consideration of environmental and psychosocial issues and the judicious use of medications. It will necessitate as well the training of nurse's aides and nurses to recognize and manage mental disorders. Essentially, a complete revision of the nursing home industry will be needed to provide the standards of modern psychiatric care for patients in nursing homes.

In Alzheimer's disease and other dementias, both physical and psychological perspectives are needed to advance care for patients and families. Each perspective illuminates a different aspect of the disease, and both perspectives complete the clinical picture.

An exclusively psychological approach misinterprets the early signs of dementia as evidence of a psychological conflict and holds the patient responsible. This may often produce unnecessary pain and delays in the adjustments families need to make. An exclusively neurological approach, while perhaps providing an accurate diagnosis, may ignore the psychological and psychiatric needs of the victim and his family.

A psychological perspective recognizes the individuality of the person with disease, appreciates his interests, likes and dislikes, and engenders empathy with his distress. It encourages caretakers to enter the person's mental experiences as best they can, to understand his experiences, and then to design approaches to improve the quality of his life. The physical perspective identifies the signs and symptoms characteristic of a particular disease and brings us swiftly to a diagnosis. The advantage here is the recognition that dementia is caused by the consequence of specific diseases, such as Alzheimer's disease or Binswanger's disease, and is not an inevitable consequence of aging. Although the cures for these diseases are unknown, the fundamental concept that dementia is associated with disease brings confidence that these diseases will eventually be prevented and cured in the way that other diseases have been: as a result of epidemiological, clinical, and laboratory research.

A treatment approach that includes both perspectives facilitates accurate diagnosis and the ongoing provision of care, not only for the patient, but for the family as well. Such care includes support and practical advice, and referral to community and legal resources. In this way, the physician works not only with diseased brains but with distressed persons. Until a cure is found for Alzheimer's disease, these principles constitute the standard of care for patients and their families.

But also, until we do find cures, millions of families will experience what the Doernbergs have. Myrna Doernberg's story is valuable because the questions she raises so frankly—Does he know something's the matter? How long will he still recognize me or remember my name? Can I help him? Is this my fault? Will his disease destroy me too? Is this inherited? Will he die?—are questions families frequently ask. Beyond posing these questions, this book expresses the pain of living with a demented loved one and asks us to question what it means to be human. Furthermore, it demands of professionals and legislators that they learn more about dementing diseases and guarantee the care patients and their families need.

PREFACE

In August 1982 I began to keep a journal. Initially it was a documentation of changes that were taking place. Ray was different, but did not perceive himself as such. Seen as isolated incidents, the changes often seemed small and insignificant. But layered one over the other they began to gnaw away at his life and relationships. Although the journal was started as an account of single events, it gradually evolved into something much more and became the foundation of this book.

I kept the journal for a year and a half. Even though I had never kept a journal before, I felt a compulsive need to record what was happening. I knew that in time I would do something with my notes. I needed to share what I had experienced and perhaps learned. I needed to do it so that others could understand what had really happened and what it was like.

The following is a true, chronological account. Most of the names have been changed, particularly those of the medical professionals Ray consulted. Specific incidents have been recorded accurately. There has been no attempt to embellish or exploit the story or characters in an effort to enhance the reader's interest.

The dialogue is composed, for the most part, of verbatim conversations between Ray and me that I either recorded in my journal as they occurred or transcribed from tapes. Frightening changes were happening in Ray's mind and in his language. I needed to preserve and someday understand those changes. I felt that by recording what he said I would eventually gain some insight. Perhaps parts of the puzzle would fall into place.

I have consciously tried not to project hindsight into this story, but rather to allow the reader to experience as much as possible the day-to-day progression as I did. My purpose is to reflect the richness and detail, but also the ambiguity and paradoxical emptiness of Ray's and my daily life.

There was no one point that I could identify as the beginning, no real turning point. It was only in retrospect that the progression became apparent. It is only through reflection that I have come to understand. Yet, there still remain unanswered questions.

It has been difficult for me to write such a personal account, exposing my feelings, mistakes, frustrations, pain, and personal, sometimes selfish, needs. I hope, too, that the love and commitment of this shared ordeal will find their equal place.

I have frequently asked myself what Ray would have thought of this venture. Much soul-searching has led me to believe that through this account Ray will touch the lives and hearts of people who otherwise would never know of the kind of suffering he had to endure. I believe he would have wanted to help others understand the insidious and relentless nature of progressive, irreversible brain deterioration and its cruel and devastating effects on victims' loved ones. I believe he would not only have approved, but would also have encouraged me in this effort.

If there is a book in each of us, this is mine.

Myrna Doernberg

STOLEN MIND

ONE

Something was happening to Ray. For the past month he had been having a number of rather alarming problems. I didn't know what was wrong, but I did know that something terribly frightening was happening. There had really been something different for a long time. Now, however, there was a pervasive quality to it. Whatever was wrong had invaded Ray's life. No longer were they subtle, isolated changes attributable to a momentary condition or difference of perception. Ray was in trouble, and I could no longer bury my head in the sand.

I called Dr. Mark Weise, a neuropsychologist, at his home one evening. I had audited a course that Dr. Weise taught a few years earlier and had also heard him lecture on a couple of occasions. "I don't know what's wrong with my husband," I remember saying. "But I feel it's either something psychological or neurological."

An architectural designer, Ray had a perspective drawing to do for work. He had been trying to work on it but just couldn't accomplish anything. After sitting at his drawing board for two days, unable to begin, he woke one morning to tell me he couldn't face work. It was the beginning of the long Labor Day weekend of 1982; Ray thought that by the time he returned to work on the following Tuesday he would have a drawing. He just needed to get away from the pressure, needed to feel more relaxed. It would all come back.

It was unthinkable to me that, at forty-six, Ray could have trouble with a perspective drawing—the first of many unthinkable things that were to come over the next year and a half that would gradually unravel and destroy our life together, a life that we had come to think of as protected by special charms of good fortune and love. Ray had worked as an architectural designer for the past seventeen years. He had graduated from Brooklyn College as a history major in the late fifties with an eye toward attending law school. But he had not felt ready for the demands involved in the case approach of Brooklyn Law School.

He was uncomfortable speaking in front of large groups and was terrified that this would be required should he enter such a program. It had taken Ray three tries to pass speech in college. Each time it was his turn to give a speech explaining how to do something, he would cut class and never show again. But because it was a required course for graduation, he finally mustered enough courage to explain the bow and arrow, props and all. He facetiously told me that he was convinced that his instructor gave him a "B" because of the direction in which he pointed the arrow when demonstrating its use.

Graduating with a history major and a political science minor, Ray was at a loss about what to do next in his life. Although he had received an excellent liberal arts background, he had no job skills. In addition, he looked so young he wasn't sure any employer would take him seriously. (When I met him, he was twenty-three, but he looked all of sixteen.) It was only after returning to school, attending Pratt Institute and studying arcnitectural design for a second degree, that Ray began to gain confidence. He felt that his portfolio spoke for him, that it introduced him as a talented, competent designer rather than the "kid" he looked like. Throughout his career Ray relied on his visual presentations to make the initial impact on clients. Even though he developed poise and confidence, delivering articulate and well thought-through verbal presentations, that large black portfolio and roll of drawings under his arm were always there for the extra support.

But now Ray couldn't remember how to do a perspective. He went to the library and took out a stack of books on perspective drawing. I couldn't fathom how he didn't remember how to do a drawing that had seemed effortless for him. When we had lived

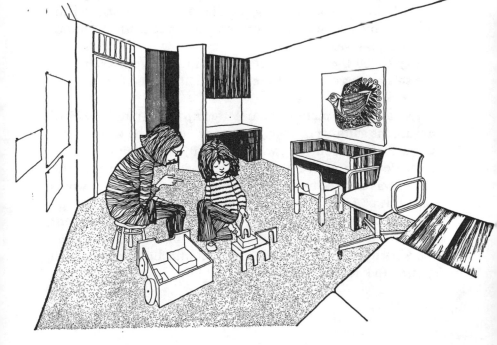

Ray drew these designs for a children's psychiatric clinic in the mid-1970s. Perspective drawing was a specialty of his, and he taught classes in it from time to time. By August 1982, however, he had forgotten how to draw this kind of picture.

in New Haven Ray had taught a class in perspective drawing. In fact he had started to write a book on it while he had been teaching as an adjunct instructor. But now he was spending hours trying to understand how to begin. He kept telling me that he felt he was so close, that he almost had it, but just couldn't remember. When I'd walk by the room I would see him at the drawing board just staring at the blank paper.

Ray stayed home from work Thursday and Friday, attempting to work without making any progress at all. On Saturday morning, I called a friend who gave me the name of an architect who also taught a class in perspective drawing. Ray called him. That afternoon, the architect came to our house and attempted to teach Ray how to set up a mechanical drawing. I could hear the two of them upstairs. The architect did most of the talking, but every once in a while I would hear Ray say "Uh huh" or "Okay," as if he were understanding what Dick was saying. Perhaps things were beginning to click. But when the architect left, Ray found he still didn't know where to begin.

Sunday morning, Ray tried again; but soon he found other things to do to avoid sitting down to what was a frustrating and overwhelming task. In retrospect it is surprising he wasn't panicked by his inability to remember. He was concerned, but not frightened. I was.

Ray called the architect and asked him to come again, and the scenario was repeated. He just couldn't remember.

Ray and I had met at a summer camp in upstate New York during the summer of 1959. I was nineteen and he was twenty-three. He was about 5'6", with dark hair, slight, but with a full face. He spoke with a New York accent; being from the Midwest I was amused by his addition of a final "r" sound to words like "idea." He was amused by my inability to alter the "a" sound when saying something like "Harry is hairy." We spent our days off together at nearby lakes, eating some "non-camp" food, betting our few dollars at the Monticello Racetrack, and getting to know one another.

In a letter to a friend that summer Ray wrote:

"I didn't have a chance to say much on the telephone last Friday, but you can probably gather, I am in love—again. Only this time it's different. I think we feel the same about each other. I know it's the best thing that's ever happened to me. She's 19, a junior at Wayne State University. She is going to work with the blind when she graduates—lives in Detroit (only bad news of deal). Thinks Ray is smartest person ever . . . thinks one day I will wake up and think she's an idiot. 5'3", 110 pounds, short dark hair, dark eyes, nice figure. You must meet her. We will be in New York for a few weeks. I will make sure you do.

"We are both afraid of this love idea . . . We are at a point where we can admit being in love, but do not like to think of all the implications—she goes back to Detroit in September—my future uncertain.

"She says she never felt this way about anyone before. First time for her—not me—but more intense this time than ever before. She wants to be sure before she admits to herself—looking for sign from heaven or something. But now doesn't look so much—accepts on let's-see basis. That's fine with me. Could possibly marry her if I were able."

We married in April 1960 and lived in Brooklyn. I transferred from Wayne State to Brooklyn College, changing my major to elementary education since an undergraduate degree was not offered in education for the blind. Ray got a job with Skidmore, Owings and Merrill, a large architectural firm in New York.

Marriage was more than I ever dreamed it would be. Somehow we never experienced that "period of adjustment." It was easy. More than anything in the world we wanted to be happy with each other. Nothing was quite as important. Our one-room, prewar, rent-controlled apartment in Brighton Beach was ample—better yet, cheap. Our lives were full—long drives in the country, an occasional weekend camping trip, movies, the beach, which was only a few blocks from our apartment, weekend trips to Deer Park on Long Island to visit Ray's boyhood friend Warren and his wife Goldie.

I always felt special because Ray loved me. The fact that someone as unique, perceptive, and gifted as he could value me must make me a worthwhile person. Not much of a testimony to my own self-esteem, but nevertheless, that belief was an important ingredient in my own personal growth. We liked being together and were aware that we had a relationship most married people never knew. I, for one, never took it for granted.

Ray entered Pratt when I graduated from Brooklyn College and began to teach in 1962. We moved from the third to the fifth floor of our building where we now lived in palatial splendor, boasting a one-bedroom apartment.

Our first child, Michael, was born in 1964. Ray didn't seem to take as much interest in my pregnancy as I would have liked, but his response to Michael upon his birth more than made up for it. A proud papa he was—their birthdays being the same day made it all that more special. Michael was a wonderful first baby—easy to please and happy. With Ray in school full-time and a new baby, we were poor, but more than fulfilled.

Ray, and often two of his classmates, Matt and Eleanor, would work on projects in our apartment. It was not unusual for our few rooms to be filled with a couple of drafting boards, cardboard scraps, press type, mechanical drawings, blueprints. They worked late into the night—and frequently all night. Often Ray would work in our bedroom, which we had partitioned into a master bedroom, a nursery, and a work area for Ray.

I worked as a substitute teacher two days a week. Ray worked part-time and for a couple of summers writing detective magazine stories. Part of his job was to comb the *New York Daily News* for stories that he could develop into fictionalized, sensationalized accounts for detective magazine buffs. Sex and gore were the two primary ingredients for a good detective story.

When Ray graduated from Pratt in 1965 he worked for a large design firm in New York. He enjoyed his job and liked the people with whom he worked. Ray loved the city and I had grown to love it too, but we could not afford to take full advantage of what it had to offer, nor could we afford to buy a house within reasonable commuting distance. When Ray got an offer from a fellow worker to join in opening their own firm in New Haven, Connecticut, the three of us (I was already pregnant with our second child) moved to Connecticut in July 1967.

David was born that summer. Small, agile, and alert, he seemed to do everything early. The four of us thrived in Connecticut. Our garden apartment on Long Island Sound was surrounded by grass, trees, the beach, and other young couples with children.

After a year in business Ray bought out his partner. Word spread, and following a few lean years his reputation for quality work brought some major jobs into the office—health maintenance organizations, hospitals, a child guidance clinic, a nursing home addition and renovation.

In 1972 we were able to buy a condominium in Cheshire, Connecticut—a small bedroom community between New Haven and Hartford. David started school and Michael entered third grade. The kids were happy—they liked school, made friends, and developed interests. Michael joined a swim team and, as he got older, played soccer. David could entertain himself for hours with Legos, blocks, and GI Joes. It seemed that he also learned to draw before he could write and appeared to have interests and talents similar to Ray's.

I continued to teach as I had throughout our marriage. Although I could never quite put my finger on why teaching was so fulfilling for me, I found I enjoyed being with and caring about my kids. Teaching made me feel good, and for the most part, I think I made my kids feel the same way.

I had started my career in Bedford Stuyvesant and Coney Island in Brooklyn, teaching third and fifth grades. As a naive, idealistic kid from Detroit, I was not ready for the street-wise, inner-city kids that I was supposed to teach. But I learned, mostly under fire. When Michael was born, I began to work as a substitute teacher two days a week. Good discipline was the key to being a successful substitute. I remember preparing for the day by getting myself into the role of a "real teacher." I learned to put up a tough exterior, modeling my facial expressions after my own sixth-grade teacher, Miss Springer. I was surprised that the kids didn't see through the act. I became P.S. 270's dependable "Super Sub." If they only had known how scared I really was!

I did some homebound teaching in New Haven after David was born, which rekindled my interest in working with special children. In September 1969 I began to do some substitute teaching at the Elizabeth Ives School for emotionally disturbed and neurologically impaired children, later accepting a full-time position.

Ives is a small private school, and there was something about the atmosphere there that fostered respect and dignity for children, in spite of any emotional or learning problems they might present. It was an environment in which everyone was nourished, staff and children alike. I found the rewards immeasurable, personally and professionally. I learned something about kids and teaching that I believe made me a fuller, more sensitive, and stronger person. It was during this period that I returned to school, earning a master's degree in special education with a concentration in learning disabilities.

Ray built bunk beds for the boys, which took him six months, as I remember. He was a perfectionist; I think he thought that someday the beds would be displayed in the Museum of Modern Art. Ray also served on the condominium association board of directors, and in his spare time finished our basement, putting up sheetrock walls, a ceiling, and track lighting, as well as designing some built-in furniture.

When did things change? What were the signs? Less initiative perhaps, some loss of interest. It was around the time Ray turned forty; maybe five or six years earlier. We had joked a little about Ray's going through a "mid-life crisis." He seemed discontent, less involved. We thought it temporary, a response to life changes. We were happy. Life was good.

In 1978, Ray closed his own office. He was tired of being his own boss, looking for work, taking care of the business aspects of his own corporation, and having periods of feast and famine. He went to work as design director for a medium-sized architectural firm in Hartford, but he knew that to be a transitional position.

There had been a change in Ray during that time. He was reading very little. He was quieter and less involved socially, lacked a certain zest for life, and didn't seem as involved in work. He had begun to lose interest in many of the things that had brought him enjoyment. He wrestled with the day-to-day concern about work and made conscientious attempts to establish a place for himself in the office. But he was unable to do so. Something was slowly eroding our lives; maybe the signs eluded both of us.

In the spring of 1979, Ray received a call from Eleanor, his old Pratt classmate. Both Ray and I had known Eleanor well. She had been a hard-working, eager, and talented student who spent hours with Ray discussing and arguing design philosophy, social issues, religion, and politics.

Eleanor had regarded Ray as her mentor. He was a few years older than the other students in his class, having already received a degree from Brooklyn College. Ray had read extensively and had opened up to Eleanor a new world.

After graduation, Ray had lost contact with Eleanor, but we had heard that she married and was in partnership with her husband, the two of them running their own firm in North Carolina. Now she and her husband invited him to join their firm, Design, Inc., as a vice-president. He was ready.

We moved to Winston-Salem in 1979, buying an eighteen-year-old, four-bedroom, brick-and-shingle split-level house. It had a large lawn in front and back; we spent endless hours in the fall raking leaves from the huge oaks behind the house.

Michael entered tenth grade and David the seventh. The boys made friends quickly, got involved in after-school activities, and came to love the atmosphere of this small, sophisticated Southern city. I went to work for the public school system in the fall of 1979, assigned as a learning-disabilities resource teacher for two elementary schools. It was the first time I had worked in a setting that allowed me to see a few children for regular periods each day and to focus on building academic skills. At Ives, I had spent much of my time on behavioral and emotional problems; this was a welcome change.

I liked Winston-Salem ("Winston" to its residents) much more than Ray. He missed being near "the city"—New York—and eagerly looked forward to his trips there on business. But Winston was a center of accessible cultural activity—unusually so for a city its size. We took advantage of some of these things—but not as much as I would have liked. We spent time at school soccer matches, going to movies, and shopping—but we didn't seem to get involved with the community or make friends, as we had in the past. Ray didn't seem particularly interested; I didn't pursue it.

But Ray knew something was still wrong; he sought help from a local psychiatrist. The doctor recommended that Ray try group counseling, since he felt he might be helped by some behavioral changes.

Ray became a part of a Gestalt therapy group. He remained in the group for about a year and a half, and although he felt support and trust from the other members, he never really was able to identify what was happening or how he could make changes. He started to go less frequently.

The group's leader ran marathon weekend sessions every few months and Ray attended one. I found it strange that Ray wanted to go. Even his involvement with group therapy was unlike Ray. He was not a person who found it easy to expose feelings to a group of strangers. He approached problems much more analytically and cautiously. But he was so anxious to make changes and feel good again that he tried things that were alien to his nature.

He drove down with two women to a house the group had rented in Myrtle Beach, South Carolina. They left Friday afternoon and were to return Sunday.

Ray called me Saturday morning. He had gone to a pay-station phone, partly because there was no phone in the house, and also because he didn't want people in the group to know he had called. After all, it had only been a few hours and he was already calling his wife. It wasn't as if we were never apart. Ray traveled frequently with his job, sometimes spending two to three days at a time in New York. But this was different. What Ray liked best was being with his family. He had gone on this weekend because he hoped it would help him, but he would have much preferred to be with us.

It was good to hear his voice. He said he missed me and wished I could be there with him. The beach was deserted because it was off-season and he would love it if we could be there together. I knew what he meant. We liked being with each other more than anyone else. We had good and close friends, but in the end it was Ray and me, and we seemed never to tire of each other.

Ray returned to the psychiatrist who had referred him to group therapy. The entire family even attended one session, at which the doctor for some reason asked his own wife to sit in. But it did not help. Things were no better and Ray knew it.

Ray was eager to be part of Design, Inc. He felt he would work on quality jobs, be valued for his skills and expertise, and feel like an important member of a team. But that never happened. From the beginning Ray never seemed to be able to perform in the way Eleanor had expected. Although, as students, Ray and Eleanor had had mutual respect and appreciation for each other's strengths, Ray's strengths were rarely visible anymore.

He did not perceive his functioning as particularly poor. But he did know that he was always afraid. In the past he had been able to confront problems in his work, but now he found them overwhelming. He found the office exceedingly stressful and demanding. He put in long hours, which he didn't mind, but found that nothing was ever good enough. He didn't know why, but he found Eleanor intimidating, and just wished she would leave him alone.

This was not the Ray I knew. It was not the Ray that Eleanor had known either. Ray had been a problem-solver. He had been able to analyze and synthesize information, getting to the core of a problem. He had been able to present a rational, intelligent case for his position. By nature intuitive and creative, he had loved design challenges and had possessed an intellectual curiosity that I admired and envied. He had always been articulate and thoughtful. People had listened and responded to him, and they had respected him.

But no one in the office got to see that Ray. No one knew the Ray who told great stories, had a marvelous sense of humor, and knew how to have a good time. No one knew the Ray who patiently helped and shared his talent, who thrived on new challenges, new projects. The Ray they knew was passive and seemed unwilling or unable to follow through on his everyday responsibilities. As one co-worker described him, "He seemed to have his head in the clouds."

Ray had worked at Design, Inc. for two and a half years. He was heading up a major job in New York City that was about to come to completion. Eleanor had had some concerns in the past months regarding Ray's leadership and follow-up. At his best, Ray would never have functioned like Eleanor. She came on strong, making threats and demands in order to get something accomplished. Ray's approach was more low-key.

In February 1982, seven months earlier, Eleanor had called Ray at home one evening. He had been home sick and was not yet feeling well. I was in the next room, but could hear Eleanor's screaming voice echoing through the phone. She was in a rage at Ray's mishandling of the project. Ray remained composed throughout the conversation, trying to calm her. But it was to no avail. Eleanor had had it. She told Ray he was no longer to be project manager on this job, a job Ray had worked on for almost two years, a job he was proud of, that was near completion and about to be photographed.

His heart was broken. He felt that it wasn't fair. He was to relinquish the project to someone who had worked under him, and to return to the office demoted. His self-esteem, which had already waned, was further reduced. It was a turning point. Ray did not know what to do.

Ray's self-esteem never improved. I would give him daily pep talks about "showing them." "You're as good or better than anyone there, Honey. Go in and show them. You have nothing to lose. Be the person you know you can be. Demand the respect you deserve by giving them what they want. Be the man Eleanor remembers and respected. I know you can do it." I believed that he could change, but that the stresses and demands were so overwhelming that he couldn't perform. He tried. He went in each day and tried, but it was never any good. His ego was destroyed.

While Ray was having problems with his "Labor Day Drawing" he also seemed disoriented with reference to time and day. He often misread his watch and generally seemed to lack a sense of time. One Sunday afternoon shortly before Labor Day, for example, Ray and I decided to attend a 5 P.M. meeting of Amnesty International. We planned to eat out afterward, since Michael was starting at North Carolina State that fall and would be leaving in a couple of days. Ray called the restaurant and made reservations for 6 P.M. He did not understand how we could not go to a five o'clock meeting, pick up the kids, and get to dinner at six. He asked me to tell him what would be a more suitable time for the dinner reservations. I know he never understood.

The next week, Ray and I planned to take one of our cars to a dealership to be serviced; then I was to drive Ray to work. We left at the same time that morning and headed for the dealership, only ten minutes from our home. I arrived first and waited for Ray. After a few minutes I began to get anxious. I waited a while longer and then asked to use a phone. I called home and then I telephoned Ray's office. He wasn't at either place. Where could he be?

It was obvious to one of the employees how distraught I was.

He asked if it would help if we retraced Ray's route. At least that was better than just waiting. He drove toward our house while my eyes darted from one side of the road to the other, looking for an accident, a stalled car, something to let me know where he was. But in my heart I really did not expect to see him.

We got back to the dealership. It had been over an hour since Ray had left our house that morning. As we drove in I saw Ray's car. When he saw me he got out of the car but just stood there. I started to cry. He laughed a little, a kind of embarrassed "It's not so bad" laugh. He didn't seem to quite understand why I was so upset. He told me that he had been lost. He said that he knew where he was, but did not know how to get where he wanted to go.

On a trip to Hawaii the previous July, Ray had left his glasses everywhere. I thought he was just not paying attention. But other incidents occurred that deep within me stirred feelings of trepidation. On the same trip, we took a cab one morning; the fare came to four dollars. Ray gave the driver a five-dollar bill, and when the driver handed him a dollar bill as change, Ray put it in his pocket. The driver was furious and Ray was visibly upset. He told me later that he did not know how or what to tip. Why was such a simple task so confusing?

After that disastrous Labor Day weekend, I related some of these experiences to Dr. Weise, the neuropsychologist. Ray had become increasingly quiet, generally passive in his response to life. He hardly ever spoke or seemed interested in anything. We had always been able to share everything; it was a relationship I cherished and knew was rare and special. We were best friends. But now I felt alone. He seemed unconcerned about what was happening in his and our life. He answered with a mere "yes" or "no," hardly ever initiating a conversation. I fluctuated from feeling that I was exaggerating to being angry and frustrated that he was abdicating from life. I felt that work was just so stressful and demanding that Ray had opted not to cope with the pressure. If he couldn't function, demands would not be made of him. I realized that gradually Ray had relinquished more and more decision-making and responsibility to me. What did all this mean? What was happening?

Dr. Weise saw Ray on September 9, 1982. In his practice, Dr. Weise studies how brain injuries and disorders affect behavior and personality. He uses a battery of tests to distinguish between emotional and organic problems. He wanted to give Ray some tests and perhaps recommend treatment.

Ray called me at home late that afternoon from the doctor's office: Dr. Weise wanted to speak with us that day. Ray picked me up, and we sat in the waiting room for a few minutes before Dr. Weise came out and asked to see me alone. He told me that Ray belonged in the hospital immediately.

Dr. Weise had given Ray various assessment tests, including a Wechsler Adult Intelligence Scale (Revised) test to determine his verbal and performance ability. The testing indicated that Ray was functioning at a level well below what one would have expected. His verbal score was 113, and the subtest scores were so "scattered" that he presented a very atypical picture. His vocabulary and information scores were high, while his memory for numbers, ability to do arithmetic, and comprehension were below average.

The performance section of the test—designed to measure visual and spatial skills—was worse. Ninety to 110 is considered to be the average range. Ray's performance IQ had dropped to seventy-nine. It was no wonder that he was having so much difficulty with performance-based tasks.

Dr. Weise noted that various psychological or physiological problems could be at the root of Ray's loss of intellectual functioning, the most probable being depression. This was statistically more likely than any other possibility, although other causes such as toxins, degenerative diseases, or metabolic disorders could account for this significant loss.

Ray's medical history posed a number of unanswered questions. At age nine he was diagnosed as having rheumatic fever, which left him with a heart murmur. After this, he began to experience severe pains in his shoulders, knees, and the soles of his feet. The cold tile on the bathroom floor was often the only relief for the burning sensation in his feet.

By the time I met him he no longer had pain in his feet. But the pain in his shoulders persisted. He would describe the burning sensation to be like hanging from a chinning bar for a long period of time. Sometimes the pain would be so severe that his hands would become very hot. I could feel the heat through a heavy sweater. Aspirin was his only relief.

In the mid-seventies Ray experienced such severe discomfort that his doctor began prescribing anti-inflammatory drugs. In the past three to four years, Ray had been taking Darvocet N, an analgesic, almost daily. It allowed him to function with little or no pain. But Ray was well aware that prolonged use could be habit-forming and lead to serious side-effects.

Recently Ray had had some problems with his kidneys. In May 1982, four months earlier, his feet and ankles had begun to swell. Several doctors recommended a kidney biopsy. My brother-in-law, a physician in Boston, wanted Ray to come to Boston because he felt that the nephrology department in the hospital with which he was affiliated was exceptional. Ray went.

Ray was to be in Boston for about five days and in the hospital two or three of those. He planned to stay with my sister and brother-in-law the rest of the time. He rented a car so that he could drive to their house. But the first night he got there, he called me from a hotel. He did not know how to get to my sister's house and instead had gone to the nearest hotel.

As far as I know, there were no other problems, but my sister said that when Ray did finally get to their house, she was aware of how reticently and passively he behaved.

The kidney biopsy indicated that Ray had analgesic nephritis, a disease caused by the heavy use of painkillers over a period of years. For some strange reason, two months prior to the symptoms of the kidney problem, Ray stopped having shoulder pains. The nephrologist had been optimistic. He told Ray that, unlike other kidney disease, this could improve and stabilize if he refrained from use of all forms of analgesics. Ray had followed this advice and had been free of symptoms. His blood pressure remained within normal limits, and he did not experience any swelling.

In October 1981, the right side of Ray's body had gone numb. A neurologist had given him a CAT (computerized axial tomography) scan and a waking EEG to determine if there were any neurological problems. The results of both tests were found to be normal. He was then given a prescription for Persantine, which he took for a short period of time to improve the circulation in his brain. The follow-up letter from the consulting neurologist to our family physician stated that Ray's case should be monitored. But nothing else had been done. Was there a problem then? Couldn't they see it?

I had read about Alzheimer's disease and asked Dr. Weise about that as a possibility. He said that it was conceivable, but unlikely because of Ray's age.

Dr. Weise called Ray in and told him generally what he had told me. Ray did not seem particularly concerned or upset. I thought he may have felt a certain relief. Now he would get some help.

Dr. Simon Hillary, a psychiatrist, joined us, and Dr. Weise introduced him as the physician whom he would recommend to handle Ray's case.

Ray and I sat and listened again to the proposal that he be immediately hospitalized. An accurate diagnosis needed to be made. How long? Two to four weeks. An eternity! I thought a couple of days, but two to four weeks—in a psychiatric ward? Ray wasn't crazy. I didn't even think he was depressed. He didn't stare into space all day, seem dejected or discouraged. It was true that he didn't function well, that he was having trouble concentrating and remembering. But couldn't stress cause the symptoms? Couldn't he really control it?

The admission papers had been filled out. It was up to us. Scary as it was, what alternative did we have? I trusted Dr. Weise.

Something was happening to Ray, and as much as I wanted to deny it, we had to find out what it was. That's what the rational part of me knew. But the rest of me was in shock. The thought of the psychiatric ward flashed a swarm of negative images before me—"One Flew Over the Cuckoo's Nest," "The Snake Pit." Ray and I hung on to each other as we walked with Dr. Weise down the long corridor to the admitting office. We assured each other we were lucky to finally get some help. I told Ray, as I had thousands of times before, how I loved him. Now I added that I knew he would be okay. How I wanted to believe that!

That very afternoon, Ray was admitted to the Psychiatric Care Unit (PCU), the psychiatric ward. When the admitting clerk asked me to sign for financial responsibility, Ray refused. He said that *he* would be financially responsible. He seemed very confident and self-assured. I had hardly seen that from him lately. I knew he'd be himself again. He needed help, some time, but it was still there. He was still the person I admired and valued so.

We went up to the ward on the elevator. It was a locked ward. Someone at the nurses' station controlled the elevator for anyone leaving the floor. The unit was set up with hotel—rather than hospital-type—rooms, each occupied by two patients. The large day room in which the patients spent most of their time was next to the nurses' station. Chairs were arranged around small and large tables. There were a couple of seating areas, a pool table, piano, and television. A refrigerator stocked with drinks and snacks was at the side of the room. A telephone for the use of patients was in the hall.

A nurse took Ray's blood pressure, height, and weight. She answered my questions and told us some of the rules. "Patients are not allowed to have anything made of glass. No lighters or matches are allowed. Cigarettes are to be kept in the day room." She pointed out the lighters that were attached to the walls for patients who smoked. Sensing my anxiety, I'm sure, she assured us that the environment was very supportive and that Ray would be fine. I felt my legs start to give way under me and my body weaken in spite of her attempt to allay my fears. I leaned against a wall fearing I might faint. I couldn't believe that this was happening. I wanted to scream, "Ray is not suicidal. You don't have to protect him. He's not going to hurt himself. He wants to live! He's different from the others here. He's special. You'll see!"

Experiencing both apprehension and relief, I went home to get Ray the clothing and toiletries he would need. It was somewhat comforting to know that he would wear street clothes while in the PCU. It would be easier for me to visit if the surroundings were not quite so much like that of a hospital. I gathered together about a week's supply of clothing and returned to the hospital about 9 : 30 that evening.

Ray was in the day room. He was quiet and appeared calm and comfortable in this setting. I was somewhat surprised. I was so tense, so frightened by what was happening. He seemed almost untouched by the experience. No questions. No spoken concerns or fears. I didn't understand.

While I had been gone Ray had talked to one of the psychiatric residents who had taken some medical history. Visiting hours were over. Ray seemed adjusted. I didn't stay long. I told myself that I was doing what had to be done. But inside I was panicked. I couldn't sort out fear from blame, from guilt, from hope.

There haven't been many nights in my life that I haven't slept, but that was one of them. I was confused and frightened. I telephoned friends and family I knew I could count on. Jan, Martha, Bill and Pam, friends in Winston-Salem where we had only lived three years; Lily and Rich in Minneapolis; Warren and Goldie in San Diego; my parents in West Palm Beach.

I went to work the next day, barely able to concentrate. It was the beginning of the school year, and I was just getting to know my new kids. It was an important time of the year for all of us, but it was hard to keep my mind on what was going on.

After school, I went back to the hospital. Ray was allowed to move around the hospital freely or even leave the hospital itself. All he had to do was sign out at the desk.

On Saturday I came to pick Ray up for the weekend. I noted that he had two forms that he was asked to sign before leaving. He signed the first one and then returned the pen the nurse had given him. He had forgotten about the second form. His movements were tentative, and he seemed insecure and unsure of himself.

During Ray's weekend at home, he became upset when faced with a small task that he could not perform—tearing off a piece of toweling from the paper towel roll, making a cup of coffee, opening a can of juice. He'd look to me as if I would provide a solution. I felt that I should not do things for him. If I started to do everything, he'd become more passive and soon incapable of doing anything. Ray did not perceive any of the problems to be as severe as I did. In fact, he denied that he was passive, lacked initiative, and was non-communicative. Never before had we viewed things so differently. Why were our perspectives so conflicting?

Saturday afternoon Ray took David, now fifteen, and some of his friends to Street Scene, an outdoor festival of craft booths and entertainment set up in downtown Winston-Salem. Ray had no trouble getting there and back. In the past two months he'd often pass the street, house, or exit for which he was looking. His judgment seemed off, and sometimes I was really scared driving with him. I was driving more and more, but felt if I overdid it, it would make matters worse. I didn't want Ray to feel I didn't trust him. He seemed to have lost enough self-esteem. Perhaps I was exaggerating this too. Ray was a good driver. I was just overly cautious and concerned. But David was surprised, too, at how well Ray did that afternoon. Why was he capable sometimes and not at other times? Could he really handle things when he chose to?

There was lots of bickering that weekend, not our usual way of interacting. It all seemed to center on Ray's not completing or even attempting to do the things that needed to be done. He didn't seem to know or care what was going on. I would give a litany of complaints. Ray would deny. Nothing got resolved, and I felt angry and exploited. It wasn't fair that he should just bow out and leave all responsibility to me. I had begun to realize that over the past months, maybe longer, I had become responsible for the entire household: managing our money, paying our bills, repairing and cleaning the house, working on the lawn, cooking, shopping, staying in touch with the kids. Ray had relinquished it all to me, and he didn't even seem concerned. What was wrong with him? He could snap out of it if he really wanted to. Couldn't he? But how could I get him to realize that? I was convinced that if he didn't make some decisions about regaining control of his life soon, he would destroy himself. He'd destroy us.

Before Ray went back to the hospital Sunday night we talked, and agreed that we could not let what was happening to us get worse by allowing friction and anger to exist between us. We needed to stick together. The doctors would find out what was wrong. We'd make it. At this point, that was good enough for me.

Ray had been in the hospital less than a week when Michael called from school one evening and asked to speak with his father. He had written a paper for his English class about his memories of Brooklyn, and he wanted to read it to Ray. I had decided that there was no point in telling Michael about Ray just yet, so I told Michael that Ray was asleep. Michael read the paper to me. My eyes filled with tears, and I imagined his did too. A few days later Michael called again. I couldn't keep what had happened from him any longer. He was not surprised. He had known something was wrong.

Ray's first week or so in the hospital was to be a time when he could be observed with all pressures removed. He talked to a psychiatrist daily, but nothing much happened. The nurses watched to see how he interacted with staff and patients, how much time he spent in his room, in the day room, and how much he slept. After a few days Dr. Hillary told me that Ray was a gifted person. It made me feel good to know that that was still apparent despite how much Ray appeared to have lost. Dr. Hillary said that it was too early to give a diagnosis, but that whatever had happened to Ray was severe.

I kept in touch with Ray's office during his hospital stay. The secretary was concerned about what she should tell the staff. She was uncomfortable with letting people know the facts and instead decided to say that Ray had taken a leave and was undergoing some testing.

But people in the office knew something was wrong. A week before Ray entered the hospital Karen, a co-worker, had called me from the office. She told me some very strange things were going on. Ray had forgotten how to run the blueprint machine. He didn't remember how to use his scale. He couldn't make a phone call without first checking with her on the questions he was supposed to ask. I had known of problems at home and knew that he was having difficulties at work, but never thought them to be of such proportions and so apparent.

Two days before he entered the hospital Eleanor, Ray's boss, confirmed my worst fears. She asked Ray to take a leave of absence. Ray wasn't functioning. She thought that he was deeply depressed. It had been getting gradually worse and had now reached a point where others were doing Ray's work. He just couldn't perform.

Although Ray was shattered by Eleanor's decision to take him off a major job and now to force a leave of absence, he felt there was little justification for either action. He was crushed, but could not understand or resolve what had occurred at the office. It was something he spoke of often in the hospital, trying to understand.

The pieces were coming together. How he had managed to function even as well as he had amazed me. With a performance IQ of seventy-nine it was surprising that he had hung on as long as he had. His relative verbal strengths helped him cover up, but he must have been experiencing frustration and fear at his inability to perform. He had talked about it some. He would say he felt paralyzed at work, didn't know how to begin. He said he would sometimes stare out the window at work and be frightened by not being able to work. But at the same time he would deny that he was not functioning. What was wrong with him?

TWO

Ray's stay in the psychiatric care unit stretched from two weeks into five. He entered on September 9 and was discharged on October 14. The doctors sent us home with a diagnosis and a lot of hope. But Ray's problem didn't improve during his hospital stay.

After a week in the unit, Ray met a fellow patient named Veronica, an attractive pianist in her late forties who had gravitated to Ray. A few days after they met, I was coming up on the elevator to visit Ray when I met one of the nurses. She told me that Ray had lost his "at lib" privileges—his freedom to move about the hospital by merely signing off the floor. He had left the hospital that afternoon and come back with a six-pack of beer under his arm for Veronica. He had come out of the elevator and walked toward the day room making no attempt to conceal it. I guess he never thought that he should not have brought it into the hospital. Of course it was confiscated.

At first Ray did not mention the incident to me. When he did, he acted as if the hospital staff were making a big deal out of nothing. He was concerned about getting his privileges back and was intent on straightening it out with Dr. Hillary; but he seemed unconcerned about the incident itself. Under normal circumstances Ray's behavior would not have been construed as unusual. But he was in a hospital, and had brought beer for a patient who was under treatment and medication. Somehow he couldn't recognize how poor his judgment had been.

Initially Ray was described in the hospital records as "quiet and reclusive," displaying "slightly blunted" or "flat and dull" affect. As time passed, however, the records mentioned his pleasant and cooperative behavior, light emotional responses, and increased emotional interaction with other patients and the staff.

Nonetheless, Ray had trouble with simple tasks more and more often. One day he tried to call me at the school where I worked. He couldn't look up the number and had to ask a nurse for help. He knew the alphabet by rote but did not know where an individual letter belonged when it was out of sequence. He had problems making a cup of coffee, making a bed, using a can opener. He couldn't figure change or write a check without a tremendous mental effort.

One Saturday morning I went to the hospital to pick Ray up for the weekend. We had planned to meet outside. Ray was not there when I arrived. I waited awhile and then went up to his unit. He had been up, but had gone back to bed. I knew he had been having some trouble with time, but I found it hard to believe that he could have forgotten I was coming.

Dr. Hillary scheduled us to see a family therapist who was affiliated with the hospital. I began to wonder if the therapist would decide that our marriage was a sham and that my perception of it was distorted. I felt terribly vulnerable, afraid that I would discover I was somehow responsible for what had happened. What if I had fostered weakness and dependence in Ray because I needed to be strong and controlling? I had always believed in our relationship; but what was happening was such an enigma that I began to wonder if our very closeness might not be a contributing factor—maybe the root of the problem.

We met with Dr. Jason Hudson, the family therapist, about ten days after Ray entered the hospital. Up until then no one in the hospital had really wanted to listen to me. Ray was the patient. But because of Ray's difficulty remembering and expressing himself, I felt that I should give the doctors information they might not get from him. I was afraid to impose myself, however, since I might be viewed as being a pushy, domineering woman.

I knew that the opposite was true. I had been forced into the role I now played because of circumstance and necessity. I had to be Ray's advocate because he couldn't speak for himself. But I feared I would be misunderstood.

Dr. Hudson was a tall, trim, pleasant man in his mid-thirties. The three of us sat around a small glass coffee table while he observed and commented. I had a difficult time understanding what he was trying to tell us. He rarely made direct statements, speaking instead in clues about what he observed. I found myself checking to see if I understood what he was saying. I would ask: "Do you mean . . . ?" "Are you saying . . . ?" I needed specific, concrete information; instead, I felt that I was being tested, trying to learn the secret that only he knew.

During the first session, in spite of difficulty, we did learn that Jason saw Ray and me being consumed by Ray's "problem." He said that I played right into Ray's hands. Ray was not weak and fragile; he was really strong and quite controlling. He knew that I would handle everything if he didn't, and in a way that was very responsible. He put me in charge and knew that I would do my job.

Jason asked Ray to think about how else he could "show his competencies" other than through his symptoms. He also asked us to describe what our lives and relationship would be like if not centered around the issues about which we were concerned. He felt that even if Ray's illness proved to be organic, our immersion in this problem was somehow useful to us. Although he said he sensed no malice or intent to hurt each other, he suggested that for things to improve, our responses to each other would have to be different.

The next Saturday I went to pick Ray up at 11 A.M. for a noon haircut appointment. When I got to the hospital Ray wasn't waiting outside as we had planned. I waited downstairs for a half hour, getting more and more upset and angry. This was the second time. How could he be so irresponsible? Should I go upstairs again? Should I leave? My instinct was to go up to the unit, but I thought about our most recent session with Jason Hudson. Shouldn't I help Ray be more responsible for himself? I left—and cried all the way home. Ray would never have done that to me. I told myself it was for his own good. In the long run it would help. I had to begin somewhere.

At our second session the next week, Jason told us that Ray dismissed whatever I said. He solicited my advice and listened to it, but really paid no attention. Ray said that he valued what I said, but he acknowledged that to follow through on things that I suggested took "too much effort."

Jason saw our relationship as that of assertive therapist/resistant patient, self-reliant wife/dependent husband. It didn't matter what words were used to describe it; we cooperated with each other in this "game." Needless to say, we were disturbed by Jason's assessment. How had things changed so? Yes, there had been times over the years when he was weak and I was strong. But there were times when I needed to lean and depend on him. What had happened to us?

Before we left, Jason gave us an assignment. Ray was to get one hundred pennies, and during the next week or so, he was to pay me a penny every time he solicited my advice or help. I, in turn, was to take a penny from him any time I found myself advising or helping him. I found the assignment ridiculous, but I grasped for any straw that might help. Occasionally we remembered the pennies and did some exchanging, but the facts were that Ray was not aware of when he asked for or needed help or direction. It was a futile and unnecessary exercise. I knew what was going on, but nothing I did could change it. When I did not intercede, by responding to or helping Ray, he was unable to carry through on tasks.

I never knew how Ray would be when I got to the hospital each afternoon. Sometimes he appeared relatively alert, and I would begin to feel hopeful. He would talk about the many decisions he would have to make, but his attitude was positive. He was primarily concerned about going back to the the office. He hoped he could be valuable again, but he also wondered if he even wanted to go back to Design, Inc. It was a high-pressure, demanding office doing quality work, but lacking warmth and closeness.

47

But even when things seemed better, Ray had difficulty with his memory—and he knew it. He told me that he was often unable to recall what he wanted to say; instead, he would select alternative, often less precise ways of expressing an idea or thought. Sometimes there were exaggerated pauses in his rate of speech while he tried to remember what he wanted to say. He said that he was afraid of trying new things for fear he would fail. He avoided things that would "stretch his mind," and got impatient when he couldn't grasp things quickly.

For years, Ray had expressed his feelings by drawing "nebbish" cartoons—line drawings of the drab, insignificant-looking character created by cartoonist Herb Gardner. His rendition of the pathetic, lumpy little figure could often convey a message better than words.

Now, Ray wanted to draw the nebbish with a Budweiser can in his hand as a reminder of the aborted attempt to smuggle beer onto the ward. I watched him as he struggled to work on it at the hospital one evening. He was able to draw the nebbish with some difficulty, but he finally gave up because he could not concentrate long enough to do the Budweiser logo.

During his weeks in the hospital, Ray made sincere attempts to alter his responses and take a more active role in our lives. He did well for a brief period of time, but he couldn't sustain the attempt.

One weekend Ray agreed to mow the lawn. He went outside, got the mower out of the garage, filled it with gasoline, and started it. Then he attempted to guide it up one row and down another. As I watched I could see that he was not able to orient himself to do the job efficiently. Every step seemed like a major task. He missed patches of lawn. Michael was home that weekend; after watching Ray for a few minutes, he offered to finish the lawn.

When Ray came in I told him that I thought Michael had volunteered to help because Ray acted helpless. I pointed out that people often volunteered to aid him because he appeared inept. Didn't he see how this worked to his advantage in that he got out of doing unpleasant tasks? Others were always there to bail him out. It had happened at work and was happening at home. Ray was struck by this observation and commented that he was not aware of it.

I found that most of the people in the psychiatric ward did not fit my stereotypes. Many were people who coped with life and functioned most of the time. Some were in crisis situations, others had periodic setbacks and needed to be hospitalized. The hospital really did provide a supportive environment, as much because of the relationships formed between patients as any psychiatric therapy or medication a patient might be receiving. Patients told their stories and shared their deepest feelings with people who were virtual strangers.

In the hospital Ray made friends with two young women and a man. They would often comment to him that they didn't know why he was there.

After a couple of weeks Dr. Hillary told me that Ray exhibited some symptoms of depression, such as difficulty concentrating and lack of energy and initiative. But he did not have other characteristic symptoms. If Ray was depressed, it was an unusual case of depression. Nonetheless, Dr. Hillary decided to try an antidepressant called Desyrel.

I began to sense that the doctors were confused. Although Ray couldn't remember a lot of what they talked about during sessions, there didn't seem to be any focus, any direction. They couldn't seem to put their finger on Ray's problem. The Desyrel was an attempt to deal with the symptoms, but the etiology remained a mystery.

One morning Ray woke up with slurred speech and a numb left hand and tongue. This was reminiscent of the time he had gone to our family doctor a year earlier. Then, the numbness was on the right side of his body, involving his right leg and the right side of his head. Dr. Hillary felt that the numbness Ray was experiencing periodically might bear some relationship to his present symptoms. He wanted to know more.

One of Ray's early symptoms was his inability to read. It was not that he could no longer read words and sentences, but that he could not concentrate well enough to comprehend what he read. He still bought books and went to the library. But they piled up unread. It had been a long time since Ray had actually read a book. He continued to read short magazine articles, but he couldn't get through anything lengthy. He missed reading very much and believed, as I did, that it was but another sign of severe stress. Once Dr. Hillary asked him how he would know that he was getting well. Ray answered, "When I start reading again."

Ray had been an avid reader, mostly of nonfiction. He was the kind of person who became interested in a subject and devoured everything on it in print. One of the first conversations Ray and I had was about bullfighting. As he diagrammed the action in the dirt with a twig, I could almost visualize the spectacle: the banderilleros with their barbed darts preparing the bull for the kill; the mounted picadors on their padded horses carrying long lances.

Where was the Ray who loved and was excited by life? What had happened to him?

As Ray's hospital stay drew to a close, I found myself reluctant to have him come home without a diagnosis. We were in desperate need of help. We couldn't be turned loose without some support and direction. But no one seemed to know what was happening.

What did Ray's low ability testing mean in terms of the future? Was he unable to concentrate and remember because of severe stress? Was he experiencing some kind of mental block that protected him from dealing with overwhelming demands? The doctors did not believe that there was any evidence of either, but they offered no other explanation. If his ability level didn't improve, how could he possibly get well and function? How could he be planning to work?

But both of us somehow clung to the belief that Ray would become the vital person I had known and needed so desperately.

We saw Jason Hudson for a third time. I was feeling hopeful. Ray seemed to have a bit more energy and was trying hard to think ahead. He seemed stronger, more assertive, more confident. I told Jason about it while we waited for Ray. Fifteen minutes later, he arrived; he had gotten lost looking for the office.

It was to be our last session. Jason noted that he rarely saw a couple who cared about and were as sensitive to each other's needs and feelings as we were. But, he said, I would need to stop protecting Ray, watching him, checking on him, always asking how he was doing. I think he was telling me to stop living Ray's life. But I didn't really think he understood how much of an investment and stake I had in Ray. I couldn't separate myself. I told myself that this was happening to Ray, not me. It was his life. But I couldn't let go. What was happening to him *was* happening to me. He was part of my soul, my being. He knew everything about me, and I knew he would have stuck by me.

Before we left, Jason said that in the future he would be willing to see me alone, or Ray and me as a couple, but not Ray alone. He did not explain his reasoning, and I didn't ask. But I resented his offer. I had sensed throughout our sessions that he blamed Ray for what was happening. Even though I had done my share of faulting Ray, my allegiance to him was so strong that I could not tolerate it from another. I also wondered how I had suddenly become a candidate for treatment. All I wanted was my husband back. I knew then that I had no intentions of seeing Dr. Hudson again.

In early October—after Ray had been in the hospital a month—the doctors decided to take a CAT scan. This is a computerized technique that uses low-level X-rays to generate a three-dimensional image of the brain. Dr. Hillary had not been able to identify a psychological basis for Ray's symptoms, and the Desyrel had not been effective. So Dr. Hillary decided to pursue an alternative diagnosis. He was concerned about the numbness that Ray had experienced in the past year and had not ruled out an organic cause.

Ray and I were in the hospital cafeteria the day after the CAT scan was done. Dr. Hillary came over to our table and sat down. He told us that the results of the scan, when compared to the one a year earlier, indicated that there might be excess fluid in Ray's brain. He did not know what it meant and thought it might have even been a misreading. A neurologist had been called in on the case. He would read the scan and see Ray the next morning.

The neurologist was Dr. Gerald Townsend, who had seen Ray about three years earlier. At that time Ray had been taking pain-killers for the undiagnosed pains in his shoulder; Dr. Townsend had strongly encouraged Ray to stop. For some unknown reason, about a year later, the pain had gradually faded to almost nothing.

Dr. Townsend examined Ray the next morning, then told us that he believed Ray had some excess fluid in his brain, probably due to the kidney problem that had been identified about six months earlier. He believed that in time Ray's body would heal itself and that as the fluid in his brain was absorbed, Ray's mental functioning would return to normal. He said that Ray seemed nutritionally deficient and would need to take vitamins, eat more nutritious meals, and begin an exercise program. He encouraged Ray to test and push himself and plan to return to work. Dr. Townsend felt that Ray's spatial skills had not returned because of a mental block.

I couldn't believe what I was hearing. Ray was going to be all right! Dr. Townsend put his arms around Ray and me and hugged us. He reassured us that with proper diet and exercise Ray would be well again.

Two days before Ray's discharge from the hospital, Ray was given vitamin injections. He was to continue taking vitamin pills at home. Dr. Townsend said we should not expect to see any improvement for at least two to four weeks. I desperately wanted to believe the good news, but I still felt a gnawing worry. I think Dr. Hillary shared my concern. No one else had seen anything in Ray's blood work-up to indicate metabolic problems. Hospital records noted that there were no signs of deficiencies.

If that were true, how would vitamins correct anything? When I asked Dr. Hillary, he said that he was trusting in Dr. Townsend's expertise. He was a psychiatrist and had not been involved in physical medicine for over ten years.

Dr. Townsend also said that Ray could return to work. I didn't see how, and neither did Dr. Weise or Dr. Hillary. Ray's functioning had not improved at all. Whom was I to believe? I could hardly rely on my own instincts. I was too close to be objective. So I believed what I wanted to believe. Dr. Townsend said Ray would be well. We'd go home and follow his advice. We'd give it a month, maybe longer. What other choice did we have?

THREE

In the hospital, Ray had talked about trying to see if he could do some free-lance work from the office as a way to test himself. He also thought he should get a résumé together. Perhaps a different job, a new place, a new beginning, less pressure.

But once at home, he couldn't even bring himself to try to draw. When we had first moved to Winston-Salem Ray had built a drafting table, which he set up in our bedroom. He had worked there at night and sometimes on the weekends. But after his return from the hospital, he never went to the board. His excuse was that it was too cold in our room. But I think he was afraid. He didn't return to Design, Inc. and began spending his days at home, alone, while I went to work.

Ray did call his office to ask for free-lance work. There was none. He began going to the library to check professional journals, looking for new openings. He still could not understand that he was unable to work at his old job, and he was particularly crushed when he saw his old job listed in the classified advertisements of one of the journals.

I decided that I would have to work at not viewing Ray as helpless. I resolved not to leave him notes and reminders when I left for work, call to check on him, or question him about what he had accomplished that day. He would have to take responsibility for getting well himself.

But my resolve was short-lived. I would commit myself to a plan of action and find I couldn't carry through. And so I was constantly torn between being angry at Ray for not doing something and feeling that I should provide the support and help I knew he needed.

I despised what I was feeling toward Ray. I was losing respect for him and found I sometimes even hated him. He didn't seem to care. He wasn't even trying to help himself.

Ray took no interest in any aspect of our lives. Financially, we were reduced to my teacher's income. We had applied for Social Security disability, but there was a five-month waiting period. Before we could qualify for Social Security benefits, we needed to prove that Ray's condition would last at least a year. Michael was in his first year of college and Ray was without any income. How long could we manage? But Ray was not concerned.

I became disturbed about how to handle the frustration and anger I began to feel. Anger was an emotion I did not experience very often, and when I did, it was for short spurts. Usually, I was able to confront the source of my anger and resolve it. Always, I had been able to talk with Ray about it, whether it was directed at him or not. But now I couldn't, and I feared that it would build inside of me and manifest itself in ways that would be unproductive and torturous for me and those I cared for. Daily there were small examples of Ray's not doing, Ray's not caring, Ray's not giving.

In an attempt to follow Dr. Hudson's and Dr. Hillary's advice I would try to find things for which Ray could be responsible. I would leave the garbage in the kitchen for Ray to take out. But there it would sit. Dishes that I would put on the counter after removing them from the dishwasher would still be there when I got home from work. It was as if Ray didn't even see them.

One evening after dinner, less than a week after his release from the hospital, Ray took two dishes off the kitchen table, then picked up his coffee, and headed to the den. I made a comment about really being tired, and he acknowledged that he had heard me with a word and a nod, but did not offer to help clean the kitchen. I knew that even if I asked him outright to help, he wouldn't. He might have said he would, but in the end I would wind up in the kitchen.

One afternoon David called Ray to pick him up from a friend's home. Ray went to get him, but after a short while he came back and told me he couldn't find him. I called David again, got the directions, and went to get him. Ray couldn't even do a simple task like picking up David.

My journal became my focus during those infuriating and frustrating times. There I could record my anger and fear. There I asked the hundreds of questions. Eventually I would find answers to most of them.

October 19

When I got home from school at five, Ray was putting anti-freeze in the car. I know that earlier in the afternoon he had met with a man who had called him about solar heating. I can't, for the life of me, figure out why Ray would let a salesman come to talk to him about solar heating. Our house is situated in such a way that even if the more than ten oak trees in our backyard were removed, we are not candidates for solar heating. Besides, of all that is going on in his life, I would think that that would be the last thing on which he would want to spend time.

October 21

After school today Ray and I started to talk. I'm not sure about the progression it took, but we ended up screaming at each other. I said that he had no resolve, no plan, no fight. It's as if he's waiting for it all to happen to him. He seems so passive. He hasn't even put his clothes away that he brought home from the hospital. Yesterday he went to the Social Security office, but didn't bring any of the materials he needed with him. He's so disorganized. He often waits for the mail, opens it, glances at it, but never seems to know or care what it is.

Ray said that he thought I had given up. He believes that he has some organic illness that is affecting his behavior. I just can't buy that. It is too convenient to blame his inertia, lack of energy, on something out of his control. I have always believed in Ray, but he is disappointing me so. I just don't know what to do anymore. Am I making it worse? I just don't know where to turn or what to do. I ask God for his help. I beg for some guidance and direction.

October 22

I was angry and upset on the way to school again today, but called Ray when I got there. "Called to just say, 'I love you,'" I told him. I don't know why. I guess, in spite of my anger I felt sorry for him, for us, for what is happening. I called again in the afternoon and asked if he would like to go to the movies with some friends. He said he would and then told me that he had just had a conversation with David. David had asked Ray if he loved him as much as he always did. Ray said that he had told David "yes," and then asked David the same question. David told Ray that he did love him, but said that he didn't respect him because he didn't think he was trying. Love and respect, he said, were different. Ray must have been very hurt by the conversation to have told it to me over the phone. I asked him if David had a point. Ray said, "No, David and you are both wrong."

One afternoon Ray and I sat down to try to set forth some goals that he could attempt to meet. We tried to establish very short-term objectives. First, I tried to get him to brainstorm with me about some projects he might try, some interests he might pursue. Ray was very passive throughout the time we sat at the kitchen table that afternoon. There were long periods of silence and I did most of the suggesting.

I had turned the tape recorder on during the time we sat there and afterward played some of it back to Ray so that he could, perhaps, see how little part he took in this attempt to help him begin to reshape his life. Ray said that he could see what I meant about his being so apathetic and unassertive. He asked that we do the same thing the next day.

There were short periods of time when I thought there was improvement. One afternoon Ray spent a couple of hours in the yard raking leaves. Sometimes he would help with part of dinner. Occasionally he would talk excitedly about plans he had and how he looked forward to getting on with his life. There were even times when he tried to work at his drawing board. Those moments always gave me renewed hope. But when they went up in smoke, I seemed to fall a bit deeper.

Ray continued to see Dr. Hillary every few weeks after he was discharged from the hospital. I knew that Ray was an enigma to Dr. Hillary. He was hopeful that the vitamin therapy would work. But I think he knew as well as I that it was much more complicated than that.

November 28

I've just about had it. I can't stand how I feel most of the time. Angry, scared, always feel like crying—knowing we're not going to make it. I've got to sort out what's happening. It's Sunday, Thanksgiving weekend. Ray has slept until eleven every morning and today until noon. I did the laundry, emptied the dishwasher, and cleaned the kitchen. He came down, put his arm around my waist and cheerfully said, "Hi, Hon. What's wrong?" I said I was just busy running around doing things. But we both knew. Right now I'm ready to throw him out! Sink or swim! I can't take it!

I realize again and again how little Ray knows about what's going on in our lives. We have a tax bill due in January, as well as Michael's tuition. I'm sure he hasn't thought of either one. I asked him yesterday if he had thought about doctors' bills and he said, "No." He has no idea of how we're doing financially and doesn't even care. I'm living and loving a memory—not the Ray I knew. That realization shatters me. If I hear "I guess so" again, I'll scream.

My being upset and angry does nothing. Encouragement does nothing. Ray does things because he's told to. He has no initiative, no drive. I hate him for destroying what we had. I don't know what to do. I just don't know what to try. I'm so lonely, so angry.

Ray had sent out a couple of his résumés, primarily to executive search agencies. His résumé was impressive. His slides of completed jobs reflected the quality of his work. In addition to having his own firm for ten years with some prominent clients, he had received a mid-career design fellowship from the National Endowment for the Arts in 1975. It was not surprising that some top firms would be interested in him.

At the end of November Ray received a call from one of the agencies to which he had written. They asked him to come to the Washington, D.C., headquarters of the agency, to interview for a job in New Jersey.

Ray had told me that I was to come to the interview. I found that strange; this was merely an initial meeting with the agency representative. But Ray was sure that my presence was required.

A couple of days before the meeting, Mr. Grail, the agency representative, called. Ray was not home. Mr. Grail asked me whether I could support a move if Ray took the New Jersey job. I assured him I could, even though I could not imagine how Ray could possibly manage any job, much less an executive position. As we talked, it also became clear that he did not expect me to attend the meeting in Washington. I did not know how Ray could have confused such a thing.

December 1

Ray tossed and turned a lot last night. I woke up and asked if he wanted me to hold him. He said, "Yes." I just caressed him in an attempt to help him relax, trying to give him the support I feel I'm not providing. After a while he reached out to make love and we both seemed to feel better afterward. When I left for school he was making coffee. We didn't talk, but I felt an affection for him that I don't feel often lately.

My new approach is going to be acceptance and support. No criticisms, implied or overt. I am going to really try and believe, as I wrote to Ray in a note this morning, that he is doing his best.

Ray went to the library the day after I wrote that entry; when he came home he said that he was really feeling down. He said that he felt things were falling apart. I knew exactly what he meant, but it was unusual for him to respond in that way lately. I realized briefly how confused and disoriented Ray really was.

And yet, I had continued to believe that perhaps he could work. Ray was to be interviewed for a top-level position when he could barely handle the minimal responsibilities of his life. Although it made little sense to me, I didn't discourage him.

Ray returned Mr. Grail's call that morning to make final arrangements. But when I asked him if his plane left from Winston-Salem or Greensboro, he didn't know. Then he told me he was to meet Mr. Grail in a lounge at the airport at 8:30 in the morning. But when I asked Ray what he planned to do after the meeting, before catching a plane home, he said he would have lunch and go back to the airport. Even when I pointed it out to him, he did not seem to understand that he would already be at the airport for the meeting.

The phone rang that evening. David answered and called Ray to the phone. All I heard Ray say was, "I don't understand." When Ray got off the phone he told me that he had agreed to go to Sugar Mountain, a ski resort about three hours from our home, at ten o'clock. But he did not remember what day he was to go, or what incentive gift they were offering for him to make the trip. When I asked why he didn't just say he wasn't interested, he said, "It happened too fast."

One afternoon a woman from the Social Security office called me at school regarding Ray's disability claim. She had called Ray and had asked him some questions. During our conversation she mentioned that Ray had had difficulty looking up my work telephone number.

The woman asked me the same questions that she had asked Ray and found conflicts in our answers. She had asked Ray if he read. He said he did. He had not read anything substantial, not even a magazine article, in months. She asked me questions about his sleeping habits, helping around the house, hobbies, self-help skills, shopping for groceries, clothing. Did he drive? How often did he get out? How did he get along with people? Did he watch television, go to the movies, take medication?

In addition to answering specific questions, I told her that his concentration was poor and that he had difficulty remembering things. I described his problems with spatial orientation, his poor judgment, general passivity, and overall inefficient functioning.

The interview really upset me. Answering those questions, one after the other, made me face how confusing life had become. Ray was not getting any better. We were only fooling ourselves; neither of us had the slightest idea of what would happen to us. I needed to call a halt to this wait-and-see approach taken by the doctors. It was time to do something.

December 2

Ray and I went to pick David up from school this afternoon. I handed Ray the keys, but he said that I should drive because I criticize his driving so much. I said that I wouldn't say anything. It is true. I am afraid to drive with Ray. His reflexes seem poor. He lacks concentration and often passes exits and streets where he is supposed to turn. But, at the same time, that is one of the few things he can still do. If I take that away from him, too, soon nothing will be left. Ray drove without much of a problem, but passed three streets where he should have turned.

On the way home we stopped at the grocery store. Ray went in. I could tell he didn't want to. He is getting a cold and doesn't seem to feel well. He was angry when he came out of the store. I asked him why he was upset. "I don't feel well and I really don't want to be walking around the store." When I asked why he didn't ask me to go in, he told me, "I shouldn't be angry at you. You didn't do anything."

Then Ray said that they didn't have any bagels, but that he had bought some Contac. David asked why he didn't remember the pizza he was going to buy. Ray answered, "I didn't want to wait on line." David reminded him that he had waited on line for the Contac. Ray responded, "So what! Big deal!" David was very hurt.

Ray was the kind of father who would have gone to as many stores as necessary to get something that one of the boys wanted. He delighted in pleasing them, indulging them a bit.

I remembered when David was old enough to ride a three-speed bike. All his friends had three-speeds, but David was small, and any bike for his size had large balloon tires. Ray searched all over to find a bike that David could ride and ended up having a bike custom-made. It was a costly investment, but one that Ray felt was money well spent.

Ray never met with Mr. Grail from the executive search agency. His cold developed into a virus. He called the morning of the appointment to cancel it, and a few days later wrote the following letter:

Dear Mr. Grail:
Please accept my sincere apologies for my failure to keep our appointment last week in Washington, D.C. Events have necessitated, at least for the next several months, changes in my career plans and goals such that I would request, at this time, that my résumé be withdrawn from consideration.
I was quite impressed by you and by the caliber of the clients you serve. I will be reactivating my efforts to connect with the design community sometime after the spring of 1982 [it would have been 1983], at which time I would very much like to resubmit my résumé for consideration.

I took Ray to the doctor because he was unable to call and make the appointment himself. He was becoming more and more dependent and didn't seem to be fighting to help himself get well. He had no idea how abandoned, afraid, and alone I felt.

In an effort to try to get Ray involved and interested in something, I managed to convince him to take a course with me at a local technical college. The course, an introduction to microcomputer programming in BASIC, began in mid-November. Driving to our third session Ray was not sure of the route and asked me a number of times where to turn. "Do I turn here? Is this it?" He was so dependent and insecure. During the session Ray yawned frequently. Even though he had the opportunity to work on the computer, as he had during the past sessions, he chose not to. He left during the session and came back to get me when it was over. On the way home he told me, "The course does bad things for my ego." I suggested that we not continue.

December 4

Ray came down to the kitchen when he got up. I was having some tea. He seemed depressed, and when I asked, acknowledged that he was. He said that there was nothing between us. I'm not sure what he meant except that I think he must feel as I do—something had changed dramatically. When I asked if it had to be that way, he said, "Yes. If it is this way, then that's the way it is." This is a recurring response. If it could be different, it would be different. If I could be different, I would be different.

Later in the afternoon I went to the library. When I got home Ray was in the den. I asked him if he felt like doing something tonight. He said he did and asked if I had checked the newspaper. It was directly in front of him, but he did not look. He just sat and watched television. I read awhile and gradually felt less and less like going because I knew we wouldn't have a good time.

I had used one of the computers at the library and told Ray that I had reserved some time for tomorrow if he was interested in coming. We could do it ourselves, at our own pace, and it was much easier than the course we had dropped. Ray didn't respond and when I asked him directly if he would like to go, he said, "No." I asked him if that meant tomorrow or ever. He said, "Ever." Damn him! Why?

Ray did go to the library with me the next day. I found the experience devastating. We started with the introductory disk, one that merely identified the keyboard. The directions were simple enough for an eight-year-old to understand, but Ray was unable to follow them. He had difficulty concentrating, but even more difficulty translating instructions into physical movements. He did not seem to be able to either comprehend a direction or hold it in his memory long enough to implement it. He was not able to find the correct key on the keyboard or to remember to push the return key after each instruction. Halfway through the lesson, he was so frustrated that he could hardly stand it. Yet he didn't give up.

I couldn't believe what I was seeing. I couldn't believe that

Ray was this impaired. How could I have blamed him for not taking hold of his life, for not fighting?

Dr. Townsend had said Ray could go back to work and, like a fool, I had believed it. Meanwhile, Ray was becoming less and less functional; but he had been trying, though I failed to perceive his efforts. He had taken on things that he knew he couldn't handle. He had allowed me to get him to take that computer course and then to try it again at the library. He had written a résumé and applied for jobs—how I'll never know.

I took the next morning off from work and went to see Dr. Hillary. We had waited long enough. Something was wrong with Ray that had not been identified.

I talked with Dr. Hillary about the past few months. I told him that something was wrong with Ray that they hadn't put their finger on. I described the scene in the library. This was not a mental block, some kind of depression (although I'm sure Ray was often depressed), something he could get over with vitamins, exercise, red meat. The more we talked, the more we began to agree on an organic basis for Ray's problem. Dr. Hillary was truly perplexed. He had relied on other experts to help with this diagnosis, but the ball was back in his court.

Although we wanted to have an update of the psychological testing done immediately, Dr. Weise wanted to wait another month so that there would be a four-month interval. Another CAT scan would be done at the same time. That meant we had to wait awhile longer.

I began to feel better; I was beginning to realize that Ray could not control what was happening. I was still frightened, but no longer angry. I wanted us to go through this together as we had everything else in our marriage. I did not want whatever was happening to divide us. But I needed him desperately and waited for the day he would come back to me . . . whole.

December 8

Ray and I took my car to the garage today. Ray was in the driver's seat when the mechanic raised the car on the lift. He had not been able to anticipate what was to happen and, consequently, remained seated. I was already out of the car and unable to help him when the mechanic told Ray to pull the emergency brake. Ray sat in the car. He couldn't find it. The mechanic told him again, but Ray just sat there. Finally, the mechanic reached up, opened the car door, and pulled the brake himself. I knew Ray must have been mortified. Later he told me, "I really felt dumb. I wanted to tell the guy, 'I'm brain damaged. I can't help it.'"

December 9

I called Ray at noon. He was filling out a job history form for Social Security. He sounded good. Our relationship is much easier now that we are both seeing the problem from the same perspective. The problem is organic in nature. Ray cannot do or help not doing. This has not stopped him from trying. In fact, he's beginning to talk about putting more structure into his life. I asked him how he felt about not working and he said, "Rootless."

Things were better between us, but the problems seemed endless. Ray got lost taking a package to UPS one afternoon. He made a couple of bank deposits one week, but didn't remember what he did with the deposit slips. Even though I tried not to get upset, I was. He felt it and told me one day, "I'm going to do better."

One afternoon in the middle of December, I met Ray and David leaving the house as I came in from work. They were going to a grocery store only a mile away. After they had been away a long time I sensed that something had happened. When they returned David reported that Ray had been in a car accident. He was making a left turn coming out of the supermarket and had misjudged the speed of the car in the lane he was to enter. He had hit the other car's rear fender and dented our front fender. David said that Ray had difficulty recording the information the other driver was giving him. He had to have it repeated four or five times. The accident wasn't serious, and it could have happened to anyone—so I told myself. But I knew better.

I told Ray that I thought that he should try not to drive as often. I tried to say it as tactfully as I could. I had been afraid of his driving for a long time, but up until this point, I'd been unable to say anything. Now I had to face it. The safety of Ray and others was at stake.

He became very angry with me and told me he would never drive with me again. He said I was a terrible driver and denied that there was any problem with his driving. He was deeply hurt and I was sorry. I cried myself to sleep that night, and I know we both slept poorly.

December 16

This morning at the parcourse [an exercise and running track] I realized that, in spite of what I'm feeling, Ray must be awfully scared himself at times. I couldn't wait to get home and just put my arms around him. I am often so involved in what I am feeling that I can't address the unspoken feelings he must have.

On the way to school I tried to put myself in Ray's place and experience what I thought he did. I found that I was feeling scared about what I couldn't do. I felt dejected and angry. I could see others as being in control and competent and it terrified me that I could not survive alone. I was becoming so helpless and dependent.

Ray continued to retain a sense of humor despite the life he was living. One morning he awoke at six to go to the grocery store. He dressed and commented, "I guess it will be safe on the roads for me to go at this hour." It was humorous, but at the same time I sensed that underneath he really meant it.

In mid-December we were invited to a party. We had hardly been out with friends for months. I missed being with other people and was looking forward to the evening. I was nervous about how Ray might come off, but was excited about going all the same. I felt that, when put to the test, Ray would be able to cover. But he must not have felt the same. As the afternoon grew on, Ray said nothing about going out that evening. It was so unlike him to do that. In the past he would have gone just because it was important to me. But as the time neared, I knew we were not going. I felt as if I were missing the prom. Maybe it was a culmination of feelings, maybe a realization of what was ahead. I don't know. But I cried my heart out.

Later in the evening Ray came to me and said he was sorry and wanted to make it up to me. He said he would invite all my friends over and have a party. He said that he felt awful. My heart went out to him. I did not understand what or why this was happening. I knew he still cared for and loved me.

December 21

At breakfast this morning the kids, Ray, and I were sitting around the table. We started talking about birthdays. Ray couldn't remember when the kids were born and he couldn't figure out what year it would have been twenty years ago. He tried to figure it out on paper, but didn't know how. He felt frustrated and I felt frightened. He knew it was simple, but he didn't know how to go about solving it.

This afternoon Ray had trouble making an egg salad sandwich. He had a hard-boiled egg in front of him, but did not know how to proceed. David tried to get him started by telling him to take a fork and mash the egg. This seemed to trigger Ray's memory sufficiently so that he could continue.

Ray wrote three Christmas cards today, but had difficulty organizing which card went into which envelope. By the third card his printing had deteriorated significantly. It was 3:05 when I asked Ray the time. He told me three or four different times. Then he stopped and seemed to be concentrating very hard. Finally, he said, "Three-o-five. That's the only way to say it. Right?"

Late in the afternoon Ray's sister called. He told her that he is much better and should be back to work in two or three months. He was misleadingly articulate and confabulated to cover the gaps in his memory. Even though much of the information he relayed was completely wrong, Ruth has no way of knowing how impaired he is.

I saw Ray cry once during all this time. It was one afternoon. Ray had been quiet all day. He had gone downstairs to be by himself; when I went to him his eyes were wet and he began to sob. He had seemed to have little response to what was happening; now the pain poured forth. He said that he was lazy, afraid to take responsibilities, afraid he would fail, afraid to commit.

I hurt for him and wondered how much of what he was feeling I had brought on. But, at the same time, I felt that perhaps this was the break that he needed. Now perhaps, in acknowledging what was happening, he could help take hold of his life, turn things around. The consequences of not confronting the problem were much worse than any effort he would have to make in getting well. He was becoming my child; dependent, without the ability to make decisions. We put our arms around one another and found comfort.

That New Year's Eve, during a party at a friend's home, Ray told me that his New Year's resolution to me would be to change things. I knew he meant it. I knew that he wanted things to be different as much as I did. I should have known then that he was telling the truth when he said that he would change, if he could.

But I believed that whatever was wrong, Ray needed to fight for his own survival. I felt that the problems he was having were much more serious than the attention he was receiving from the physicians indicated. Ray was deteriorating mentally and emotionally, and no one, other than myself and the boys, could see the proportions it had taken.

He denied and rationalized, but he was losing his hold on life. He was learning helplessness and I was fostering it. Whatever agony this brought Ray, I felt it provided him with a security and protection from a world he was afraid to face. He would sometimes tell me that to change took "too much effort." I would tell him that he was one of the brightest, most talented, gifted, and able people I had ever known, but that he was just vegetating; that if he didn't practice living a functional and productive life again, one day he would no longer know how. Even if there were a physical basis to it all, he must help himself.

But in time it would be I who would learn. I would reinterpret in retrospect the expressions of desperation and pain. I would learn what "too much effort" really meant. I would come to know about emotional shallowness, lack of judgment, responsibility, initiative, and commitment. I would come to understand why Ray couldn't fight back.

FOUR

In early January Ray was given another battery of tests, including a CAT scan and a psychological re-evaluation. We met with Dr. Weise the afternoon of the testing, before the results were known. He told us nothing that afternoon except that this was one of the most puzzling cases in which he had ever been involved. That evening and the next day, I was apprehensive about what the findings would reveal. I could not concentrate on anything. I dreaded but was anxious to hear what diagnosis they could give us.

The following day I came home after school to pick Ray up for our appointment with Dr. Weise. Ray was to meet me outside, but he wasn't there. I went in. It was getting late, but he said he was not aware of the time. I was impatient watching him move slowly, as if he didn't care or feel any urgency. We were in the car when Ray remembered that he had left his glasses in the house. He went back to get them, moving as slowly as before.

Ray waited outside while Dr. Weise reviewed the results with me. He said that most people who take two IQ tests within a short period show improvement the second time—a phenomenon psychologists call the "practice effect." But Ray's scores were no better—in fact, they were a little worse. His verbal IQ now was 109, and his performance score was seventy-four.

The CAT scan also showed no basic change. There was too much fluid in Ray's brain. Neither Dr. Weise nor Dr Hillary knew why that had not changed, and both thought it was time for Ray to see a neurosurgeon.

I asked Dr. Weise how much of Ray's condition might be psychological. "Ray gives me a strong impression that he's pulling my leg," he said. But he added that he couldn't trip Ray up, and in the end, he had concluded that Ray was not malingering, or depressed.

Ray joined us and Dr. Weise repeated his findings. Ray asked if there was any treatment. Dr. Weise told us that a neurosurgeon might recommend a "shunt"—a tube in the skull that would drain some of the excess fluid. Ray asked if it would make him any better. Dr. Weise said he did not know. The fluid might be causing Ray's problems; but it might be just a symptom of something else—"although," he added, "we have no idea what it could be."

Leaving Dr. Weise's office, I felt somewhat elated, relieved of a terrible pressure and burden. It wasn't Ray's fault. He couldn't help it. I could stop blaming him and expecting things from him. What Dr. Weise had told us was potentially bad news. A psychological disturbance could be treated. I knew that much less was known about neurological disorders. But, knowing it was organic allowed me to release the anger I felt, to stop trying so hard to change Ray. Most of all, it allowed me to accept and love him again. I had been confused these past months and had changed my perception of what was happening from hour to hour. I vacillated between thinking whatever was happening was within Ray's control and feeling that it was organic and out of his control. I had struggled with an anger I couldn't resolve or express. I hoped this was the end of that struggle.

That afternoon I felt a love for Ray that I had not experienced very often in the last months. What we were to face remained a mystery, but at least there would not be friction or conflict between us. Ray was not able to control what was happening to him. He needed me more than ever now. My perception of what had been happening began to change. I began to see how much Ray couldn't do, rather than wouldn't do. In fact, over the next few weeks, problems began to permeate everything Ray did.

One of the few things that Ray could still enjoy was watching TV. But our local cable system used a selector box, which meant that the TV itself had to be tuned in to channel 3. Ray couldn't remember that the box was the mode of channel selection, not the TV itself. Ray would change the channel on the TV, sometimes watching static for hours. Because he had so much difficulty sleeping, the TV in our room would often be on and I would hear him changing the channel, with no success, during the night.

Ray had always enjoyed cooking. In fact he probably did as much, or more, cooking than I did. He would buy *Gourmet* magazine, concoct new recipes, and delight in having us try a new dish. Patiently, he would chop, dice, baste, and sauté some of the most complicated and time-consuming recipes, enjoying the process as much as the repast. But now he was having more and more trouble remembering in what order to take simple steps. By early January Ray would ask David, who also enjoyed cooking, if he'd like to help him. The truth was that he was becoming so impaired that he needed someone to assist him. Or was it that he was assisting?

One day at the supermarket, Ray purchased groceries for more than the amount of cash he was carrying. He left the groceries at the register and came home to get the checkbook. He went back to the store, paid for the items he had purchased with a check, and then selected some additional items for which he wrote another check. Poor planning or poor memory?

Our washing machine had stopped working and, although reluctant to spend the money, I bought a new one in mid-January. At the store the clerk asked about installation. Ray very confidently said that he would install it himself. I was surprised. He couldn't make a cup of coffee, handle change, follow a recipe, or identify a car key on a chain of three keys. But if he thought he could install the washing machine, I would not deny him that. Maybe he could.

So we took the washing machine home in our little station wagon. David and a couple of his friends carried it into the laundry room, but in a minute I knew that Ray had no idea of where to begin. I had always loved to try my hand at assembling things, building, tinkering. Ray had always helped me try whatever I wanted. I always knew he'd bail me out if I got in over my head. But now I knew I was on my own. The hook-up of the washing machine was mine.

I read and followed the directions, and Ray assisted. He helped lift and hold while I fitted and tightened. Even though he understood less than I at this point, his very presence gave me the assurance I needed. It may not seem like a tremendous feat that I hooked up the washing machine, but it was one of the tests of survival that I felt I passed, one that helped with the future we were to face.

It didn't take long before the anger and frustration I thought I had put behind me reared their ugly heads. Among the most difficult things to handle were the emotional rejection and indifference I experienced from Ray. I couldn't believe that he wasn't able to do something to help himself, and save himself and me from what was becoming a progressive and pervasive destruction of not only his, but my life. I desperately needed him, but I was losing him.

January 9

I'm feeling terribly rejected by Ray. When I tell him I love him he answers that he loves me too. But it always has to be elicited. He is not demonstrative physically or verbally. He never does anything without direction. How I wish he would just take me around like he used to, hold me, appreciate me, tell me that he loves me. We made love this morning but it's so different now. There's nothing there. Sex is just an act. It's so empty and meaningless.

The other day I asked Ray if I was important to him. He said, "Yes." When I asked him why, he said, "Because I depend on you." David, sensing my ever-present need, told Ray to "hold Mommy." Ray came to me and put his arms around me. Contrived as it was, it felt good, and I pretended that I was safe again in his arms.

Over those weeks, I'd recall an incident that had happened previously and see the situation in a new light. One such memory was Ray's birthday almost one year earlier. I had seen a wood lathe on sale at Sears. Ray had always wanted a lathe. He had taught a woodworking shop at a teen camp where we had both worked years before and had loved it. I put the lathe on lay-away because I wasn't sure whether it would be worth buying. Ray had lost interest in so many things recently. Even though I knew he would love the thought of having it, I feared it might not get used. As the time grew closer and my decision to purchase it became no clearer, I told Ray what I had done and of my concern. He advised me not to buy it. I think he was afraid of the pressure I would put on him to use it if I did buy it. He was concerned that he might not and chose to avoid the problem altogether. I was heartbroken, and I think he was, too. Somewhere within him he must have known his limitations even then.

January 17

I asked Ray if he had any idea of what I wanted. He said, "Yes, but I guess I can't give you what you want." He doesn't even try. If he saw someone hurting, wouldn't he reach out with a word, a touch, something? He says I am carrying no more of a burden than he, but he does nothing. He wakes up, dresses, and sits all day. Yes, I'm angry. I know he's sick. But can't he do more than he does? Does his illness affect his feelings toward me, too? He tells me he has remained steady through this whole thing. I think he's numb, not steady. I can't live like this. I am so alone, so empty, and in such anguish. I want him to be the way he was. I need him so desperately. Ray says that things are not so bad. Why are they so bad for me?

Ray's appointment with the neurosurgeon came on January 19, 1983. He was surprisingly anxious. I wanted to go in and see Dr. Daniels with him because I didn't think he would accurately convey the problems he was having. But I didn't. I remained in the waiting room, nervously flipping through old magazines while the doctor examined and talked with Ray. When Ray came out, however, I was uncomfortable with his explanation and asked to see the doctor.

I remember the awful tearing feeling I experienced. It was one that I had felt frequently of late. I didn't know when I could trust Ray; I questioned the simple accuracy of much of what he said. I was doing the same thing now. What must he feel like? I was treating him like a child.

Dr. Daniels explained that the brain is bathed in cerebrospinal fluid. This fluid is secreted into the ventricles, or cavities, of the brain as well as the space around the brain. It is then absorbed into a membrane that surrounds the space. But Ray's brain was either producing excess fluid or not absorbing enough. So the ventricles had become enlarged, putting pressure on the brain cells. Dr. Daniels said he didn't know where the extra fluid was coming from, but that Ray had more than a normal amount of fluid in his brain. He and the radiologist had made a diagnosis of normal pressure hydrocephalus (NPH)—what used to be called "water on the brain." He recommended an operation to insert a shunt that would let excess fluid flow into Ray's abdomen. But the operation offered at best a slim chance. Studies had shown that people with "idiopathic" NPH, that is, NPH without a clearly understood cause, were less likely to show improvement than other cases of hydrocephalus. Dr. Daniels gave Ray less than a 25 percent chance for improvement. But he could offer no other treatment as an alternative.

"Usually," he explained, "NPH has a triad of symptoms: progressive mental deterioration, walking imbalance, and incontinence." But Ray's only symptom was mental deterioration— dementia. I felt that his walk had changed, too. It wasn't the wide-stance gait that I had read about, but rather a stiff, slow walk with a bit of a shuffle. It wasn't dramatic enough for the doctor to pick up, perhaps, but I could see it wasn't the quickstepped bounce that he had had previously.

Ray and I were both upset when we left Dr. Daniels's office. We knew his chances were dim for recovery even with a shunt, but we were offered no other options.

January 19

Ray gets upset with me because I cry so much. I do look like I fall apart, but I'm also always thinking about what I can do, learn, read. He feels I'm back to my old position of somehow making him responsible and wanting him to make the best of what he has, wanting him to fight. He's right. What other choice does he have? I cry, and beg, and question. Why us? What have we ever done to hurt anyone? Why give us such a happy, fulfilling life and then take it away?

I know that I am no better than my neighbor who is plagued with problems, but I find I feel cheated and angry. At the same time I hold on to believing that this will end, that we will have our good life back again. I know I am hanging on to an impossible dream. I must live for today. Maybe I will lose that, too.

Ray had been getting chest and leg spasms for about a year. On our numerous trips to the emergency room for the chest spasms, we were unable to learn what the cause of the problem might be. But the spasms continued, lasting anywhere from two to twenty minutes. Were these spasms related to damage caused by the rheumatic fever Ray had as a child? What about his heart murmur? It had not interfered with his activity in any way for years and could only be heard after exercise. But now the doctors said the murmur could be heard even at rest.

Dr. Jerry Elwood, a cardiologist, was called into the case. He explained that Ray had originally had a "first-degree" heart-block, a condition in which the electrical impulses that regulate the heartbeat move through the heart more slowly. Now it had become a more serious second-degree block. This could cause potential problems during surgery. It was decided that it would be necessary to perform a heart catheterization before the shunt operation. In this operation, surgeons would insert a tube into Ray's femoral artery at the groin, then thread it up to the heart to take measurements of the pressure. The catheterization would show whether Ray would need a pacemaker, either temporarily or permanently. Dr. Elwood also cautioned me that other problems might be found. Because of previous damage from rheumatic fever, Ray might need a valve replacement. He might even have coronary disease. If any of these problems materialized, then surgery and recovery would postpone the insertion of the shunt.

The irony of it all was that none of this would improve the progressing dementia that existed. But without the catheterization, the neurosurgery could not be performed.

The hospital medical library became my afternoon and weekend haunt. I didn't understand half of what I read, but I felt an awesome responsibility in making a decision about a surgical procedure in which a shunt would be placed in Ray's brain. There was no alternative treatment, but with less than a 25 percent chance of its being effective, was it worth it? Although there appeared to be no alternative, I felt I owed it to Ray to make an informed decision. And so I read everything I could and spoke to people who I thought could provide some background.

Ray did not ask me anything about what was going on. Under different circumstances he would have been very involved in the decision—and openly frightened. But he did not seem particularly concerned. He didn't inquire as to what I'd learned when I would come back from the library, and when I'd volunteer information, he hardly seemed interested.

One Sunday afternoon I convinced Ray to go to the medical library with me. It was late January and I primarily wanted to get him out of the house. I parked the car about two blocks from the library. After the first block the walk became very icy. I have always been afraid of ice and experienced my usual tenseness as I attempted to negotiate the glazed surface. But Ray, who was never disturbed by ice, who would skate along, or at least walk with ease, panicked. His legs stiffened and he stopped walking. I took his arm, but he had a terrible time picking his foot up and planting it again. I had never seen him like that before. He was terrified, and it took him what seemed like a half hour to walk the one block.

January 21

Ray and I have very confusing and upsetting conversations. He feels that basically this is out of his hands, and if he sleeps late and watches TV, it really doesn't make any difference. I agree to some extent, but believe for his mental health, he should do as much as he can. My concern is a continued life of this. If a shunt is implanted and it works, he believes he will be all right; all of this will vanish and he will become functional and productive again. But what if things don't change? Is this going to be the quality of his life? He says he doesn't feel pride in himself because he isn't working. He moans and sighs a lot and when I ask him what's wrong, he says, "Nothing."

January 23

Early in the day Ray said that if I was going to the store I should get something for him. I said that I wasn't planning on going. In the evening, while I was on the telephone, he told me to get off. When I asked why, he said that it was time to go to the store. He was so anxious to go that we went even though I didn't need anything and didn't think he really knew what he wanted to buy. In the store Ray took an armful of packages off the shelf as if looking for something in particular. Then he didn't know what to do with them.

When we got home he got angry at David for no apparent reason because he didn't like what David was watching on TV. I made him a cup of coffee and asked him how it was. He said it was fine. A minute later he took another sip and said, as if it were the first time that he had tasted it, 'This is bland." He seemed to know that he was all mixed up and it tore another small piece from my heart.

How can I describe what it was like to watch someone you knew as a vital, bright, alive, alert human being die mentally in front of your eyes? Like most of the things we learn best in our lives, it can only be fully understood by those who experience it. It is one of those experiences of life that is beyond words.

As the days passed, incident upon incident suggested a progressing dementia. Often, however, Ray was able to hide behind his relatively intact social skills. As a psychologist friend of mine describes the phenomenon, he was able to "punt." But the more aware I became of his problems, the more I saw how futile were his attempts to mask his impaired state.

One day, for example, one of David's friends asked Ray who had won the Jets-Miami game. Ray couldn't remember "Miami," and so answered, "Not the Jets." It was funny and a great cover, but I wondered how often in the past he had punted and I had not known. Had he covered at work in that way? Had he covered with us at home?

Ray tried to change the linens on our bed each week, but gradually became less and less able to manage even this. One day he put two pillow cases on the same pillow. He always had trouble figuring out how to put the blankets on and even had difficulty straightening them.

January 24

When I got home from school today Ray looked especially nice. He had showered, washed his hair, and put on fresh, clean clothing. I commented on how well he looked. He did not respond to my compliment, but instead asked me if he was missing something. As he asked the question, he lifted his pant legs. He was not wearing socks. He had on shoes, but no socks. I told him that he wasn't wearing socks and he looked at me with confusion. He said he knew that he didn't have them on, but he didn't know how to get them on. I tried to explain that he would have to take his shoes off first and then put on his socks. He didn't understand. He started to talk about things I didn't understand and asked me, "Why do you have to put on so many layers in the winter?" He wasn't upset, just confused. He didn't know how to solve the problem and wasn't even sure what was wrong.

Ray has said during the past weeks that he didn't know "how to fill things." He's forgetting how to put things in logical order and sequence. This applies to thoughts, as well as physical or performance skills. The other day he held a steak in his hand. He wanted to put it in a pan, but didn't know what he needed. In another situation he didn't know to get a glass for a drink he wanted, so he attempted to pour the liquid from a pitcher into an already filled glass that he saw.

Sometimes he seems enough in touch that I think I'm exaggerating, but I can't be. I'm beginning to be afraid that he will do something dangerous. Yesterday, when I came home from school, three burners were lit on the stove. He had tried to fill the kerosene heater, but instead pumped kerosene over the garage floor. I'm also afraid of his driving and have asked David not to ask Ray to drive him anywhere. Even if he doesn't get lost, his responses are slow and inaccurate.

I talked with Ray about my concerns over some of the things that had been happening, and he agreed not to go anywhere, cook, or fill the heater until after the surgery. I hated to take away what was left of his dignity, but I was becoming very concerned about his and our safety.

January 26

Ray doesn't know what day or month it is anymore. I asked him today what month it was. He said, "November, isn't it?"

He tried to use the bank card for after-hours service but didn't know how to insert the card, push the buttons, or where to put the card when he was finished. "Where do I put this?" he asked. I told him to put it in his wallet. "What do you mean?" he questioned. I had to give a number of verbal prompts and sometimes help with the specific steps to get him to put the card away.

In mid-January, Ray was denied Social Security disability. The reason stated on the denial was, ". . . Although your condition is severe, it is not expected to remain disabling for at least twelve continuous months as the law requires. The evidence shows your condition will prevent you from doing your past job, but it will not prevent you from doing other types of work which are within your ability. It has been decided, therefore, that you are not disabled according to the Social Security Act."

There was no way Ray could do any work, no matter how menial. With the denial came information as to how we could request that Ray's case be re-examined and reconsidered. It meant submitting updated evidence within sixty days. There was not a doubt in my mind that Ray was entitled to benefits, and so I began the appeal process. It would be three months before we were able to persuade the Social Security Administration that Ray really was disabled.

I set up a telephone interview with an examiner at Social Security for one afternoon when I thought I would be available; then I had to cancel because of a time conflict. The Social Security office called anyway, and Ray took the call. I knew his answers would be, at best, vague, and at worst, totally inaccurate. I decided to go to the Social Security office and check the information Ray had given. As I expected, the answers were inaccurate by virtue of omission of the most pertinent information. I explained, as best I could, the circumstances to the woman with whom I spoke, and she allowed me to take new forms home to complete and resubmit.

On January 31, 1983—the day Ray was to enter the hospital for his heart catheterization—someone stole my purse. When I got to work that morning and realized it was missing, I called Ray at home and asked him to look for it. He put the phone down and came back to tell me he couldn't find it. I was surprised he remembered to come back to the phone. Because his memory was so poor, I was confident that it was there, but that he just didn't remember what he was looking for.

I came home early to take Ray to the hospital, and indeed the purse was nowhere to be found. I spent the next two hours calling to report the theft to the police, insurance company, credit card providers, motor vehicle bureau, etc. Ray was impatient with my state of turmoil. He did not understand why I was upset, but seemed to sense my tension. He found this threatening, and it made him feel insecure.

Ray was admitted to the hospital late that afternoon. Unlike the Ray I once knew, he was quite calm. Although he had been told why he was in the hospital, he was not able to attach his usual emotions to that knowledge. Ordinarily, he would have been very frightened and would have bombarded the doctors with questions about what, and when, things would happen. But he did none of that. He passively cooperated, but was unable to give an accurate history and did not seem to comprehend much of what the doctors did tell him.

The catheterization took place the next day. It was somewhat different than the usual procedure. In a heart catheterization, it is customary to examine the coronary arteries by injecting dye into them. But, so I had learned, the dye is a severe strain even on healthy kidneys, and it was not unusual for kidneys to stop functioning when dye was injected. The doctors worked without the dye in order to spare Ray's kidneys.

The procedure took about three hours; I tried to cross-stitch. When Ray returned, he was only mildly uncomfortable, but had to lie prone for six hours. The catheter had been inserted through the groin, and it was necessary for him to lie still so that the bleeding would stop.

Good news came that evening when the doctor told us that the preliminary study indicated no heart surgery would be necessary. No calcification or narrowing was evident in the valves. The valve problem was not significant and the block, although a second-degree one, looked benign. This meant it would not develop into a more serious, third-degree block, in which one's pulse drops to about twenty. It would not be necessary to do anything. The doctors felt that Ray would not have any trouble with the neurosurgery. It wasn't over. But at least we were over this hurdle. Ray went home that weekend anxious to leave the hospital. He was to return the following Monday.

When I picked him up to take him home that Friday afternoon, the nurse said that he had been very quiet. He was dressed, but looked terrible. He was weak, pale, and his face quite thin. He took tiny, shuffling steps as we walked down the hall to the elevator and out of the building. As we left the hospital and moved out into the cold winter air, Ray remarked that it felt good. He seemed to become more aware and alert. I knew that it was important that Ray be stronger by the time we returned to the hospital on Monday. Michael would be home that weekend; he was good at getting Ray to be somewhat more active. I knew that the stronger Ray was, the better he would handle the surgery. The Valium IV that he'd been given for the catheterization and the sleeping pills that he'd been getting at night weren't helping him either. He was docile and passive enough as it was. The drugs turned him temporarily into a zombie.

February 4

We're down to the wire now. After all these months, this is the step that we must take. A possible improvement. Perhaps a cure. I try not to think too much about the outcome, but I can't help wondering how I will handle the results. If ever I needed strength and guidance, I will need it if the surgery is not successful. I want so much to believe that I will be there for Ray, no matter what. Will I?

I noticed that our friends would call to see how Ray was, but not ask to speak to him. Sometimes I felt that he must have felt lonely and abandoned, even though he did not seem to respond. Sometimes I wanted to ask friends to call or visit him, but hesitated. It was easy to think that they couldn't handle it. But to me people's lack of personal contact with Ray chipped away a little more at what I viewed as his humanity, his dignity.

The problems with Ray surfaced just as Michael began his first year at North Carolina State University, a two-hour drive away. Michael seemed to adjust well in his first semester, but he had more difficulty in his second. He didn't find much relevance in his classes, found it difficult to commit himself to meet academic demands, and wondered if he should stay. I felt terrible that the home situation might be aggravating his difficulties; but I could not talk to Ray about my concerns.

February 5

I woke really upset and concerned about the confusion Michael is experiencing. It is his first year of college and I want to be able to provide some guidance. I felt so alone and desperately needed to talk with the only other person who really knows and understands Michael. It was about 11 A.M. when I went to Ray and asked him to please listen and try to help me. I shared some of my concerns, looking for a response on which I had become so used to depending. I needed his strength, his confidence, his wisdom. He didn't say anything. He just stared at me, oblivious to my need. I went into the bathroom and cried.

Sometimes I feel like I have a big hole in my stomach. It's open, and empty, and so painful. It aches and begs to be filled, with a touch, some sign of understanding, something that will somehow bond Ray and me again. I don't know how to make the pain go away. I feel I can never be weak, never be dependent. He isn't there for me. He doesn't know that I hurt and can't make the emptiness and loneliness go away. And, yet, he is physically there.

Desperately and continuously I attempt to stir what was. But there is an impenetrable mesh screen that keeps us from touching one another. He stands before me. He looks like the Ray I know. But he is different. Unsuccessful, frustrating, and terrifying as it is, I continue to try to reach through the mesh, hoping to reach one small piece of him.

FIVE

Ray left the hospital on February 4 and returned on Monday, February 7, for implantation of the shunt. A neurosurgical resident came in to describe the actual operation. Ray's head would be shaved and two burr holes would be made in the skull—one for a silicone catheter that would be placed in the brain, and another behind his ear where the valve would be placed. Then a tube would be connected directly to his abdominal cavity, running through an incision in Ray's stomach. The tubing would run under the scalp to the valve and allow the cerebrospinal fluid to flow from the brain, thereby relieving the pressure.

Ray listened, but did not appear particularly concerned. I didn't understand how he could care so little, be so unconcerned about something that ordinarily would have been terribly frightening. But his unnatural calm was a plus in a tense situation.

On the day of the surgery I arrived at the hospital mid-morning. Ray was a little anxious, but very quiet. The knot in my throat was getting tighter, and even though I knew this was the chance for which we were waiting, I couldn't help but be nervous. I felt we were making the only decision possible and that we were in good hands. I had read about the procedure and had been assured by two physicians in other departments of the hospital that the neurosurgeon we were using was one of "the top men in his field." Even more important, perhaps, we knew that without the surgery Ray didn't have a chance.

Ray went down to surgery about noon. Friends stayed with me in the family waiting room. We walked around the hospital, drank coffee, and tried to talk about other subjects. But the time passed slowly, and the mental image of what they were doing to Ray kept surfacing, no matter how I tried to repress it.

About three hours later, Dr. Daniels came into the waiting room. Even though I could not read anything into his facial expression, his posture, his pace—something—convinced me that it had gone well. He came over to me and most gently and kindly told me that it was over. There had not been any problems. "Now," he said, "it is time to just wait and see."

We waited down the hall from the elevator. Each time a gurney appeared, my heart pounded. I was afraid of what Ray would look like. We were there about an hour when I saw a gurney move out from the elevator hallway and head toward Ray's room.

I know that anticipation of fearful things is often worse than the reality, but, nevertheless, I approached the gurney cautiously. Only half of Ray's head had been shaved, while the other side was untouched. This made him look significantly worse than if they had shaved his entire head. His head was not wrapped in layers and layers of gauze as I had imagined. Instead, there were bandaged areas where the incisions had been made.

The elevator ride had nauseated Ray, and even before he got to the room, he was sick to his stomach. The nurse gave him an injection of Phenergan for nausea and codeine for pain. His eyes were open and, although he was still under the effects of the anesthetic, he was surprisingly aware and alert. His color was good, and his vital signs were normal.

I called the nurses' station from home twice during the night and was told that Ray was doing fine. Even though the surgery had gone well, I did not experience the relief I had expected. The surgery itself was only one step. It did not assure us of anything. Its effectiveness was yet to be known.

Ray was in the hospital seven days. In the elevator one afternoon, I met a woman who looked familiar. As we stood near each other, I remembered who she was and knew I had to speak to her. She was the wife of the psychiatrist Ray had initially gone to see when we had first moved to Winston. Ray had gone back to him about a year before. At that time the doctor suggested that he meet with our entire family. What a fiasco! The doctor's wife was at the session, which was something we had not expected. And I'm not sure what her credentials were.

Before we began, they laid out the ground rules. Everyone was allowed to say whatever they wanted without having others interrupt. I began by explaining how difficult I was finding it to live with Ray's apathy and uninvolvement. They told me I should direct my remarks to Ray. I knew it was a technique that psychiatrists use to get people to communicate with each other. But that was not difficult for us.

I started to do what they asked, but found it uncomfortable and artificial. After a minute or two of directing my words to Ray, I stopped and told them that we did not have those kinds of problems and proceeded to describe to them what was happening from my perspective. I related my frustration at trying to help Ray become more productive and at how fruitless I was finding it. I told them that no matter how I stroked, encouraged, nagged, loved, nothing worked.

David didn't say much, but Michael was eager to share his feelings about two people he loved and respected. He told the psychiatrist and his wife that he felt he could freely express his views and feelings and felt he lived in a loving home. He told them he could not ask for better parents. He described Ray as different, but excused him by stating that he was under an inordinate amount of stress from work. He talked about Ray as a father, and his words made me feel so warm. I knew how he truly loved, admired, and valued Ray.

Ray was very passive during the session. He expressed concern over what was happening, but didn't understand why he was having problems or how he could change his situation. At the time I thought it was a good session. Looking back I think it was because I looked like the good guy and had an opportunity to have people listen and see me as such a loving and "self-sacrificing" person. I guess I needed that because I was so frustrated at my inability to make changes.

But, in retrospect, I saw it as a "dump on Ray" session. In the end the psychiatrist gave Ray no direction, no encouragement. The doctor's wife summed up Ray's inability to perform by saying, "He just doesn't want to work." I believed that such a remark was supposed to make Ray suddenly become aware of how he was coming across, to prompt him to make some dramatic change in his life, to light a fire under him. But later I interpreted such a statement as insensitive and uninformed. For Ray, it must have been a knife to his already near-nil self-esteem.

Now, a year later in the hospital elevator, I asked the doctor's wife if she remembered me. She did. We got off the elevator and I told her the events of the past six months. I had to vindicate Ray in her eyes—to let her know that she had harshly misjudged him. I was feeling very angry at her, but I managed to talk normally, as if I were relating some information that might interest her.

She seemed quite surprised and interested and said that her husband would be anxious to hear what had happened. I wanted them to know that Ray was not the malingering, uncaring person they must have thought him to be. I wanted them to know. I wanted some of my guilt for having been so wrong to be relieved by vindicating him in their eyes. They were wrong! I was wrong!

Ray recovered quickly from the surgery. He was relatively free of pain, and had none of the possible after-effects to which we had been alerted. A few days after the surgery I visited him and brought a gift. I had bought a pair of new slippers that I wrapped in colorful paper. He seemed to like them. But that night, nearly midnight, Ray called me at home. I was surprised because he knew I would be asleep. Or did he? His sense of time had been quite distorted, and he did not seem to realize what hour it was. He said he had just wanted to call me because he hadn't seen me all day. My heart sank, and for the first time since the surgery I got scared again. He didn't remember that I had been there that afternoon. He didn't remember the slippers I had brought.

I had tried to be positive and strong, but now I was beginning to become overwhelmed with the potential future that we would face. It was too early to tell. But what if Ray didn't get better?

During the next few days there were other indications of Ray's confusion with time. He called me one night at ten and asked if I was ready to come at eleven. I was to pick him up at eleven—but 11 A.M. the next day. At 6:30 the next morning Ray called and asked where I was. He said he was waiting for me and was very upset that I wasn't there. I explained that the roads were very icy and that I would be there later in the morning.

He didn't understand why I wasn't there and couldn't figure out what I was saying. He said, "I'm not crazy." I changed the subject and asked him if he was going to shave. He got angry and responded, "I'm not a raving beauty." I said that I had just asked him if he was planning to shave. This time he said, "I'll see."

My heart was heavy. I was to bring Ray home from the hospital. We had had our shot at helping him get better. I was afraid to have Ray come home. I didn't know what to expect, but somehow I felt that we had more to face.

When we arrived home that morning Ray let me cut the hair on the side of his head that had not been shaven. I cut it as close to his scalp as possible so that his hair would grow in evenly. He took a shower, shaved, and emerged looking much better. Then we had a strange conversation. I'm not sure how it started, but at one point I said, "It was really insensitive of your office not to send flowers or something to show their concern." Ray answered, "I'd rather have sugar. They know how hard it is to get sugar and that's what I would really like and they should know that." It was funny, but like the other "funny" things that had happened in the past months, it was laced with a portent of tragedy.

Our family stuck together. Ray continued to get stronger physically and recovered from the surgery significantly better than I had anticipated. The boys pulled with us. They were as affectionate as ever with Ray, and more than ever to each other. We were relaxed and open about what had been happening, and were aware of the possible outcomes. Although Michael had less contact with Ray because he was going to college, the time he spent with his father was important. The boys teased and joked as they always had. It was different now, though.

February 13

Today was a hard day. I felt tremendous pressures for all of the things that I have to do. At night I watched a TV show about a woman who gave all her children away when she knew she was to die. I cried long after it was over. Unexpectedly, Ray came up to the bedroom. He put his arms around me and said, "I really believe things will be good again." I want to believe him.

There were times when I believed Ray was improving, even during those first few weeks. But I wasn't sure, and knew I just might be reaching. His thinking seemed more logical, and he seemed better able to figure out the sequence of steps involved in a task. He was able to fill the kerosene heater; he could remember how to make a cup of coffee.

One afternoon Ray and I talked about the possible future if he did get well. I knew we shouldn't. It was too early and would be too disappointing if it didn't happen. But it was so exciting to think about Ray's working—his being alert and alive again. He talked about wanting to help out with things, but didn't know where to start.

February 15

I took Ray to the emergency room tonight. He had a severe leg spasm, similar to the kind he gets in his chest. It lasted so long that we both got scared. They wouldn't let me into the room where he was, so I don't know what he told the doctor. They were not able to identify the problem and the spasm passed.

February 19

This morning about 5 A.M. Ray went to the kitchen to make a glass of chocolate milk. After a few minutes he came back upstairs. I was half-asleep and only semi-aware of what was going on. He told me he was a little confused. I tried to talk to him without really waking up to see what the problem was. I asked him if he had put the chocolate in the glass and he told me he had. I told him just to add the milk. He went downstairs and I fell back to sleep. A few minutes later he came up and said, "I'm not sure what I did. You should come and look." I knew that I'd better get up. I had been reluctant to do so, being torn between savoring that early morning sleep and the call for help that I could hear in Ray's voice.

When I got to the kitchen I saw an empty glass on the counter. I didn't know where the chocolate milk was that he had made until I saw the box of chocolate powder on the counter. When I looked in the box I saw that Ray had added milk to the almost-filled box of chocolate. He did not know what he had done. He had not realized how he had been unable to process the steps to make a glass of chocolate milk. Later, he said, "It wasn't so bad. The proportions were just off." But in his own way he was as disturbed by the incident as I was.

This afternoon Ray went to take a shower. He became very confused and wandered back and forth between the two bathrooms at least twenty times, not knowing what to do. He was very quiet and vague all day.

When I came back from the grocery store, I brought the groceries in and put them by the front door. I asked Ray to help me carry them into the kitchen. He came and seemed anxious to help, but instead of picking up a package and carrying it into the kitchen, he took one item out at a time and walked to the kitchen. He didn't comprehend why that was an inefficient way to accomplish the task.

In the evening we went with friends to see *Sophie's Choice* at the movies. I found that, as we walked from the car to the movie, I was leading and sometimes pulling Ray. He walks so stiffly and without a sense of where he's going.

I could see Ray getting worse. Every day it seemed there was something else with which he had trouble. Making a cup of coffee continued to be a monumental task. He would stand in front of the four canisters that stood on the kitchen counter and not know what to do. He would put sugar in the coffee canister instead of in a cup, or coffee in the sugar canister. My coffee and sugar canisters looked like salt and pepper shakers. One day he put twelve teaspoons of sugar in his coffee. When he tasted it, he had no complaints.

Ray still liked to go to the library, and on one occasion brought three books into the library to return them. But when he came out of the library, he had two of the books he brought to return. Somehow, instead of returning them, he had renewed them.

Always a careful smoker, Ray now became somewhat careless about dropping ashes. One day I found him dropping live ashes into a plastic trash bag.

He was showering and shaving less and less frequently. He said it was too hard. I began to see how hard it really must have been. There are so many steps involved in something as seemingly simple as shaving.

Ray knew that he wasn't getting any better. He knew he was getting worse even though the realization did not seem to penetrate or cause him the emotional pain one might have expected. He did not feel the devastation that I did. His bright, capable, alert mind was being destroyed. I couldn't believe it was happening, and the reality of it shattered me in a way I had never known.

One evening Ray watched a TV program on Alzheimer's disease. I had fallen asleep, but in the morning he told me it was a terrible disease. In watching the program, however, Ray did not seem to associate his problems with those of an Alzheimer's victim. We had cautiously considered Alzheimer's disease from the outset. But only an autopsy can provide a definitive diagnosis of Alzheimer's disease. It is a disease in which all other possible causes of dementia, many of them treatable and reversible, must be ruled out first. It is therefore often referred to as a disease of exclusion.

David began to take on more and more responsibility. He knew he was losing his dad, and in the process there was a role reversal. He seemed happy, involved and active in school, concerned about but accepting of what was happening to Ray and our family, and as loving as ever to Ray and me. When he was with his friends, though, he kept quiet about our difficulties. He did not bring friends home and avoided all situations in which Ray might have contact with them. But he and I talked. We needed each other. We were the only ones who really knew. He told me one day, "I like when Michael is home because then I feel I don't have to worry so much."

February 22

I called Ray three times from school yesterday, but he didn't remember that I had. In the evening we picked up David at a friend's home. Ray is always glad to go for a ride and still seems to have a sense of direction.

In the evening we watched a movie in which Susan Blakely played Frances Farmer. Ray told me, "That isn't Frances Farmer. That's Susan Blakely."

Lee Grant played the role of Frances Farmer's mother and when I asked Ray if she (Lee Grant) was Frances Farmer's mother, he answered, "I don't know. I have never seen Frances Farmer's mother." In an attempt to help orient him, I told him that Frances Farmer had died in 1970, but that didn't help. I asked him if he knew what year it was and he said, "It's somewhere in the sixties. 1961, I think."

He went into the kitchen to get some cheese and crackers. He took out a pitcher of juice and I gave him the crackers. Then he took a knife and headed toward the den. I told him that he still needed the cheese. He said that he had it and held up the crackers. He insisted that he had the cheese. He took two crackers out of the package and stood holding the knife, not knowing what to do. He did not realize that the cheese was missing, but knew that something was wrong. I got the cheese for him and he tried to balance the cheese and crackers unsuccessfully on his lap. I told him to get a plate from the kitchen. He came back with a cup.

The day took its toll on me and I started to cry. Ray got angry and told me to stop. My crying only adds to his confusion, but I couldn't. A few minutes later he asked me if I was crying because he was having trouble. I said, "Yes," and he told me, "Don't worry, I'll get over it."

I cried off and on all night. I'm so afraid of the future. What will Ray be like if he doesn't get better? Will he eventually have to be institutionalized or need someone with him all the time? How will I manage financially? I am overwhelmed. I long for the life we had, so loving, so close. He was my best friend. He taught me so much. I know that one of the reasons I am handling this as well as I am is because of how nurtured I was and how that nurturing allowed me to mature and grow. I ache for our life together. He was everything to me. I have always known that ultimately it was Ray and me. I love the kids with all my heart, but know that they will grow and make lives of their own. And that's as it should be. But I fear for what will happen to me.

I live with memories. The man I love is but a shell of himself. It's a tease. He is there, but not there. He is the same, and yet he is different. He is a member of our family, and yet not the same member of the family. How will I cope? How will I keep from becoming bitter, lonely, and withdrawn? What will happen to us? How will I live a life that will be fulfilling and meaningful? All I have are questions. When will I know the answers?

Over and over, I told myself I was too pessimistic. After all, it was only a few weeks since the operation. The doctors said that if there were an improvement, it wouldn't be immediate. But not only wasn't there an improvement, Ray was worse.

There were days, however, or at least parts of days when he

seemed more alert. He was always a good sport, allowing us to test his memory. It appeared that he still retained rote memory for things like multiplications facts, the days of the week, months of the year, counting. But when asked to apply this information, he drew a blank. What day is before Tuesday? He didn't know. What are the winter months? He didn't know. He did not know how old he was, how old the kids were, the grade David was in. Nothing was consistent. Sometimes he would answer correctly, but most of the time he was incorrect. Sometimes David and I laughed at his answers because they were ludicrous. But even the laughter was saturated with tears.

As memory failed Ray, he would forget in what order to put on his clothes. I would find him wearing two pairs of underwear or a wool sweater with a shirt over it. Without assistance he was at a loss as to how to help himself.

I continued to share with Ray the way I always had. Perhaps I was making it harder for him, but it was such a pattern of our life together that I felt it would be demeaning not to. Besides, I just couldn't change something that had been such an integral part of our relationship.

As the days passed and Ray encountered more problems, I felt that there was less chance for recovery. He became more and more dependent on David and me. Sometimes I felt that he did not really have normal pressure hydrocephalus. I was reading about pre-senile dementia, especially of the Alzheimer's type. The more I read, the more Ray seemed like an Alzheimer's victim. If he had Alzheimer's disease or some other irreversible and untreatable form of dementia, the future was dismal. I wanted to scream, "Stop! I can't watch and live this way any longer."

There were many logistical things to be done, in addition to the daily problems we faced. I spent a good deal of time with the paperwork necessary to qualify Ray for Social Security insurance, as well as filing for a waiver of premiums on his life insurance so that we could keep that in force, and getting his company insurance policy to continue coverage for a preexisting condition so that he would have complete medical coverage.

The times the four of us were together were few. David and I found that when Michael was home we were a family again, and his presence lightened the atmosphere. We laughed more, talked more. There were more of us who could relate.

At dinner one evening when Michael was home he commented, "We need to appreciate what Daddy can still do." David observed, "Daddy knows what he wants, but the connections aren't right." The boys went to Ray and each took an arm. They walked him over to me, and we all held each other. It was what we had come to call a "family hug."

I learned how much I needed other people. I had never needed to go outside my marriage before for strength. But now I did. I reached out and found that people responded. They cared. They listened, and they helped me gather enough strength to continue.

Ray's seemingly vacuous emotional responses were the worst things I experienced during this period. I would beg him to come back to me. I'd hold him, stroke him, tell him how much I needed and wanted him, but he was unable to respond.

Ray was usually quite docile, passive, and gentle. But on occasion, I found that he would have unexpected catastrophic reactions. One night we were walking up the steps to bed. I patted his rear in an affectionate way. He stopped and turned around angrily. He told me to stop or he'd hit me. I was shocked and then hurt. This was not the Ray I knew. He did not even realize that I was upset or how he had responded.

March 15

Ray and I had an argument tonight that ended nowhere and just hurt him. He told me, "You see everything so pessimistically. How can I get better when you're always down, have no hope, have me dead or a cretin?" I tried to explain what I saw happening; he is having so many difficulties, and I don't know how to help.

He responded, "You should just be glad I'm alive. It's a life! What's so great about your life? What do you do that's so productive?" I tried to explain that I was afraid that he'd get hurt leaving the stove burners on, turning the heat up to 90. But he minimized all of my concerns.

By the end of the conversation he was very depressed and I was in tears. He told me, "I can't hold on to what I have and it gets worse day by day." Is that what I wanted for him to feel? Part of me did. Part of me feels that if he sees what's happening, he'll start to fight to get well if that's within his power. I'm so confused. I don't know how to respond to him. He rarely talks about it, and aside from last night, does not seem upset or concerned about what's happening. Do I want Ray to see what I see? Yes, because it would help me. But, no, because it would destroy him!

We returned to see Dr. Daniels about five weeks after Ray's surgery. When I got home from school Ray was dressed, but had not showered or shaved. He went upstairs to shave before the appointment. I heard the water running for about ten minutes, but when I went into the bathroom, Ray was just standing in front of the mirror. He did not know what to do.

Dr. Daniels asked what we were seeing. I told him that there was no improvement, perhaps some deterioration. There seemed to be more problems with orientation and more overall confusion, problems ordering the individual steps to accomplish a task, some problems with dressing, and I thought there was some difficulty with word retrieval. Ray had also been experiencing numbness in his arms and face. The doctor examined Ray's eyes, took his blood pressure, and had Ray touch his nose, turn his hands, and do other simple actions. He checked his legs and feet and examined the shunt pump and the incisions—they were healing fine. He ordered a series of X-rays to make sure the shunt was working efficiently and scheduled another CAT scan and psychometric testing in two months.

When I asked Dr. Daniels about a possible prognosis, he said that it was impossible to tell. It could take any course. Ray's condition could stabilize, get better, or get worse. Ray could deteriorate quickly, or slowly. Anything was possible. "Only the Lord knows," he said. He said that Ray should try to do as much as possible—walk briskly every day, do some yard work, do chores around the house. I knew from his suggestions that he really did not understand how impaired Ray was. But we would try.

SIX

In March 1983 I went to an Alzheimer's Disease and Related Disorders support group meeting. Even though I did not know whether Ray's diagnosis of normal pressure hydrocephalus was accurate, I felt that Ray had some organic brain disease. I was anxious to meet people with whom I could talk and learn.

There were about fifty people there. We each introduced ourselves and explained our reasons for attending. I felt, from my very first contact with this group, that all those "strangers" knew and understood. They knew what I was feeling, living, and losing. I began to feel an immediate bond and intimacy with people I had just met. They were family members whose loved ones were in various stages of the disease and were either at home, often with a full-time caregiver, or had been placed in a nursing home.

A lawyer whose mother had Alzheimer's disease was the speaker. He spoke of the many problems that family members needed to deal with when a loved one becomes demented and mentally incompetent. It was very depressing to hear what he had to say. But I knew that I had to begin to make some plans.

I was working and David was in school. We were leaving Ray at home, and although I tried to avoid dealing with the situation, I knew that Ray should not be left alone. What if he fell or got hurt? He would not be able to use the telephone or get help for himself. I wasn't sure that in the event of a fire he would know to leave the house, much less call the fire department. But it tore at my heart to think that Ray needed someone to care for him. Perhaps it would have been easier if he had had a physical handicap. He needed help, though, with simple, everyday tasks: cutting his meat, tying his shoes, telling time, preparing a sandwich.

But would Ray accept a stranger in our home watching him, helping him? Would he feel degraded, demeaned, embarrassed? What would the everyday responsibilities of a caregiver be? There would be little to do, and yet someone needed to be there, ready to assist with anything that touched his failing memory. And what about David? What about me? How would we handle a stranger in our home taking care of our mentally deteriorating father and husband?

Even if I decided to go ahead with it, how could I manage financially? We were living on my teacher's salary and Social Security disability. I was afraid to touch anything in the bank, for fear I would really need it later if Ray ever had to be placed in a nursing home. Michael was in college and our expenses were far greater than our present income.

It was too much to contemplate, too overwhelming to confront. Maybe it wasn't as bad as I was making it out to be. I'd postpone any decision for a while longer. We'd go on as we were. Put it off a little longer.

Within the next month I met with a lawyer and a trust officer at the bank. I established a trust so that in the event I predeceased Ray, he and the boys would be provided for (at least for a while). I also had two new wills drawn since circumstances were quite different now. Power of attorney, I learned, was another crucial document I would need from Ray. And I, in turn, granted the trust power of attorney for me, since I felt Michael and David were still too young to have to make those financial decisions.

The power of attorney for Ray would not nave to be registered until I actually needed it, but if I waited much longer, I feared that Ray might not be considered competent. In that event, I would have to go through an expensive and lengthy guardianship procedure. I also knew that Ray felt strongly about not employing undue measures to prolong life, as I did; so I had living wills drawn for each of us.

I knew that Ray had some understanding of what I was doing, but primarily felt that he still trusted me. I explained to him much of what was going on, but his confidence in me endured far longer than his intellectual understanding of what was taking place.

Under Social Security Reconsideration, Ray was granted disability benefits in April 1983. By that time, two doctors were able to determine that his condition was probably not reversible and would not improve.

Showering and shaving continued to be problems. Ray had always been very meticulous about his appearance. He loved clothes, rarely went unshaven, and showered daily. For the past few months I found he would wear the same clothes if I didn't put them in the laundry, but he was still showering and shaving. Gradually, however, he would shower and shave less frequently, until now he would go for days without doing either.

One morning David and I convinced Ray to take a shower while we were working in the yard. We were outside quite awhile when I saw Ray standing at the front door in his shorts. All he said was, "I need help." He must have been trying to adjust the water most of the time that we were in the yard. When I got to the bathroom, there was no hot water. The faucet was running full force. Ray did not know how to turn the water off. He was noticeably frustrated and disturbed. For the first time he told me, "I want to kill myself. I can't do anything. I can't even adjust the damn water!"

Just as showering and shaving became problems, so did dressing. When we learned that Ray was unable to adjust the water, we made sure we were there to get the water adjusted and there to turn it off. But now, putting on clothing was becoming more difficult. Ray would put pants on backwards. Often when he would dress, he would forget an item of clothing completely— no shirt, no underwear, no belt, no socks. But he never knew what was missing or how to remedy the problem when it was pointed out to him. Sometimes I found him laying an article of clothing on the floor in an attempt to position it so that he could figure out how to put it on correctly.

He would wake me up in the middle of the night to change

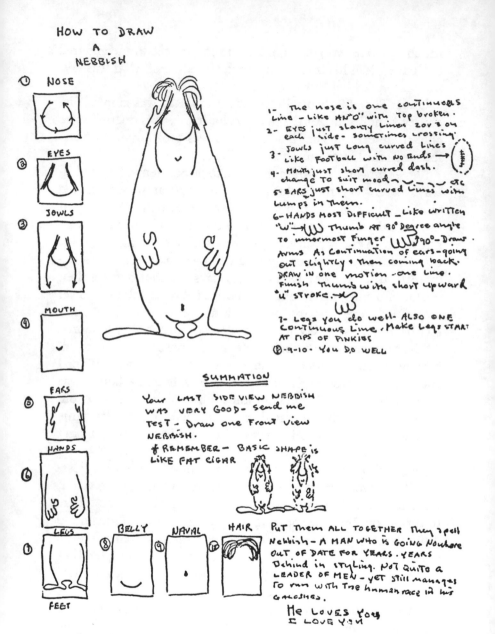

Ray adopted the Herb Gardner "nebbish" as his own symbol. He made the drawing above for Myrna. When a doctor asked him to draw a nebbish in 1983, he painstakingly produced the sketch at right.

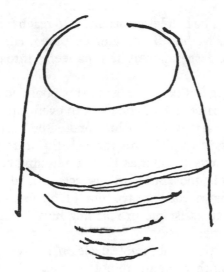

the TV channel; would sometimes smoke without using an ashtray; would try to straighten the blankets on our bed, but not know how; would try to make juice from a frozen concentrate, but not be able to get past opening the can. He would come outside to help with yard work, but found he was unable to do more than carry trash bags filled with debris to the front of the house where the city trucks would collect them.

Always testing, seeing what Ray could still do, I asked him one day if he thought he could still draw a nebbish. He said he could. He tried, but failed. He seemed depressed and told me, "You shouldn't have asked me to do that. Don't ever ask me to do that again."

March 16

I sometimes have an image of Ray in the middle of a large pool of quicksand. He is up to his waist in the mud which is gradually consuming him. He is slowly sinking and being swallowed by the earth. There is nothing onto which he can grab or hang. He is alone and unable to save himself. His arms are up over his head as he helplessly attempts to reach for someone or something to save him from being devoured. His face is lined with panic and desperation as he slips deeper into the murk, an inch at a time.

I am standing at the very edge of this pool and reach out to him to help. I can touch his hand. I can even gain a fairly good hold on the fingers of one of his hands. But I can't manage a firm enough grip to pull him through the mire that engulfs him. I extend myself as far as I can, stretching beyond what I believe are my bounds. But I am unsuccessful. I do not have the leverage or grasp needed to save him. I look about for someone or something to assist me in reaching him. There is no one. There is no thing!

I am faced with an unbearable decision. I may choose to take a step closer so that I can grab hold of him. This would bring me into the quagmire and I know that eventually I will be devoured unnecessarily with Ray. The second option is just as painful. Let go. Release the almost imperceptible hold I have. Stand by the side and watch as he is drawn deeper and deeper into darkness.

That is what I feel I am living. The choice of what I must do is clear, but difficult. Many of us die even though we live and breathe. And although pieces of me die as I lose Ray inch by inch, I know that I must make a choice. If I choose to live, I must choose to do that in the most meaningful sense of the word. My instinct is often to hold on to Ray and sink with him. He is my life, and if I am losing him, I have little left. But another part of me vies for attention. It says, "Do what you can. Try as hard as you can. Love him and protect him, care for him and value him. But do not die with him. Death need not be a physical end. There are the living dead. People who give up. People for whom there is no purpose, no meaning. Don't do that. You have much. You have a legacy of love and strength that will serve you and others." And so I struggle with a choice, the answer to which I know.

March 18

I asked David today how he was feeling lately. He told me, "I feel like I've lost a daddy. Sometimes I feel so empty."

March 20

I feel like I'm going through a denial and acceptance state at the same time. Sometimes I believe that this can't go on and that Ray will be well, even though intellectually I know there is no basis for this. But this feeling seems only to be at the surface, and right below it is a feeling of dread.

March 23

Ray showered today. I told him I was glad he did, but he denied having done it. He was so adamant that I started to doubt my own sanity for a moment.

We went to the parcourse near our house and walked something under a mile. Ray noticed that he didn't walk straight. He also seemed to shuffle his right foot. When we got back to the car Ray went to the driver's side. I asked if he was going to drive. He said, "No." But instead of walking around to the other side of the car, opened the back door, got in and then slid over to the other side. I couldn't help but laugh. Again, it was that, or cry.

Our good friend Goldie came to visit from San Diego. Her husband, Warren, was Ray's best friend when they were kids, and the three of them had known each other before I met Ray. Warren remembered Ray ("Buddy," as his friends and family called him) as a Brooklyn boy who, in Warren's words, had developed an exterior of toughness but had a softness of the soul. He would say that Ray liked to describe the skyscrapers of Manhattan as "granite walls which formed canyons as vast and deep as the Grand Canyon." This was their view of Mother Nature.

Warren remembered Ray as the second baseman on the Brighton Beach team, right end, set shooter par excellence, center for the hockey team. Warren once told me that "Bud would have been the Brighton 14th Street candidate for College Bowl. Buddy had more facts, names, general information in his brain than anyone I knew. He was a silver-tongued drugstore cowboy. He'd have been picked first for the debate team whether the argument was Yankees versus Dodgers, socialism versus capitalism (he could argue either point persuasively), or any other of life's questions of religion, economics, politics."

Ray was the fastest kid on the block, especially when it came to running from the gangs of tough kids. He was a piano player at teenage parties when they'd gather around to sing some Nat "King" Cole song or "Those Wedding Bells Are Breaking Up That Old Gang of Mine." "Bud was the creative one who could draw cartoon caricatures or execute an occasional oil painting. He had girls on his mind, but was too shy to ask them for dates. Buddy and I would sit for hours in my father's car planning dates, parties, our lives. He was the visionary who used to ask 'big questions.' 'Where does the universe end?' 'What is time and eternity?' He'd continually question life and ask, 'Why?'"

The night Goldie came we talked until three in the morning. I couldn't believe how involved and animated Ray was. I hadn't seen him like that in months. He talked about his feelings, about what was happening, and how he didn't see why this was so hard for me. He recounted his hopes for the future, which, under the circumstances, seemed strange and unrealistic to me. He was so alert and involved that I thought that Goldie must really think I was exaggerating. I knew Ray was "punting." He was behaving and responding like a person I hardly remembered.

As the days went on, however, Ray became quieter and more like the person I had been living with. Goldie could see what was happening. She was the only person, outside of Michael and David, who had been with him long enough to really understand how he had changed. He seemed to have the ability to present an acceptable social facade for a while, but was not able to hold on to it for long. During Goldie's stay a couple of revealing incidents occurred.

One day I had to do some grocery shopping. It would only take about fifteen or twenty minutes. I suggested to Ray that I drop him off at the parcourse. By the time he walked around, I would be back to pick him up. He agreed. I hurriedly picked up a few things at the grocery store and returned to the parcourse, which is on a heavily traveled road. As I came down the road, I saw Ray standing, waiting for me. He got in the car and told me he had to go home. He said he had wet his pants. It was the first time anything like that had happened. I asked why he didn't go in the woods. He said he didn't know. He was somewhat embarrassed, but not to the extent I would have expected.

One afternoon Goldie and I decided to visit a mill on the Blue Ridge Parkway. Ray and I had been there before, but I wasn't sure of the route. I commented to Goldie that I hoped I was going in the right direction when Ray quite emphatically said I was going the wrong way. I know that he hadn't been thinking about it at all, but my inflection or some momentary involvement triggered his interest. In the past, if Ray had said that in the same convincing tone, I would have turned around, since I was not feeling confident myself. And even now, knowing what I knew, I thought maybe he was right. There were times when his memory was accurate, and I could not dismiss everything he said. So I stopped and bought a map. Ray was not right, but I could see that it was taking me a long time to give up my pattern of listening and responding to him.

As the days passed I encountered more and more instances of Ray's confusion and memory loss. One morning I found him in the bathroom folding a two-foot-long piece of toilet paper; he said that it had to be put in order. Later, I found him unrolling an endless amount of toilet paper. I went to him and took his hand from the roll he was so furiously unwinding. He knew that he was confused, but he did not know why.

When he dressed, he put on two sweaters. I suggested he put a shirt on underneath, but he needed me to assist him. He was unable to put the sweater on. It was like dressing a child at an age when they have only begun to learn about extending an arm to assist someone dressing them.

Early in April, sex became a major problem. For the past year Ray had become almost as passive in lovemaking as in other aspects of his life. As Ray's memory deteriorated, as he forgot how to dress, wash, and shave, he also forgot the steps involved in making love.

Ray remained gentle, albeit passive, most of the time. But he continued to have catastrophic responses when he was frustrated by a situation he did not understand. I found that I responded as if he were the Ray I had known. I would be hurt, cry, and soon after would chastise myself. I knew I should not respond as I might have in the past, but I just couldn't help it. Ray was doing and saying things that were contrary to what I had expected and known.

One day I was in the bathroom that Ray wanted to use. He came to the door. I told him to go to the other bathroom. I knew he would not understand what to do. I couldn't even go to the bathroom. I locked the door, but he did not understand. He kept knocking on the door. Again, I told him to use the other bathroom. But he couldn't stand the frustration any longer. He told me to "shut up." He was unable to do as I had asked. I think he understood the words, but could not follow the instructions. He was conscious enough of the problem to realize that he didn't know what to do and was probably frightened at his inability. But his dependence on me was so great that my unwillingness to assist him set him adrift. He truly was unable to resolve this situation.

I knew that Ray's thinking and language were changing. Although his vocabulary seemed relatively intact, he had great difficulty organizing and maintaining a stream of thought. He often said things that seemed to make sense only to him. I was desperate to find a way to preserve what he said so that in time I would come to understand the changes and progression in his loss of thought and, subsequently, of language.

In order to do this I would need to have a record of Ray's actual words and try to capture his tone of voice, its pace, inflection, and intensity—all the nuances of language. The only way I knew to do this was to actually write down or tape-record what Ray said. Recording conversations verbatim somehow made listening and participating in confusing, upsetting conversations less difficult. I think it also allowed me to stand back a bit, feeling I was doing something valuable. I would be able to document what was happening so that it would be understood—perhaps in a new context.

Early one morning Ray asked me, "Do you know how to make up a bed?" I said that I did. He continued by telling me, "There are rules and you have to know the rules." Then he started to talk about "patterns in powder," adding that it was important to know the pattern. He spoke softly and thoughtfully, in much the same way he used to talk to me about some philosophical or sociological issue that he had been mulling over in his mind. He was patient as he always had been in trying to explain something to me. But now he made no sense.

"You know how things belong?" he asked. "It's sort of irritating to have things run against the pattern." When I asked for an example of what he meant, he said, "A sheet seems to want to go in the direction of the bed and it's irritating to have it not conform—it's disturbing to have it jumbled. We have to have things go to a point which is restful."

ME: Do things seems jumbled?

RAY: No . . . It's just in you. You know what things have to be like. You know what you have to do with the patterns.

ME: What else besides sheets have patterns?

RAY: Bedclothes, in general. No other reason for them; no function for them. They don't conform. Don't know where the rules come from. The patterns are not all that clear. Don't take it personally. All these things are subtle. They're all gray, not all that apparent. Patterns are gray on gray, blue on blue . . . You grow up with them. They're so strong.

ME: What is a pattern?

RAY: Do you know what a solid is? Well, you know a pattern. Solids and patterns work with each other. [He was pointing to our solid blue blanket.] Why did we buy this? It works for us. We seem to have an unspoken agreement about things. The sum total is our taste. You make choices in life. Most things you choose are not solid, in patterns, embossed. Most things are chosen blindly. You have to be aware of them. They're an ever-present factor in life. Some people's whole enterprise is making these choices.

Although Ray had recovered from the surgery, he sometimes complained of pains in his head. He would describe the pain as "currents that are turned on and off" or "like fluid rushing in to fill up the lobes." The doctors prescribed Tylox, a pain reliever composed of Tylenol and a derivative of codeine not metabolized through the kidneys. Within a few days, after taking the Tylox, Ray no longer complained of pain in his head. But with his failing memory, I had to be careful not to leave the pills out since he would take them.

Ray was still walking around the parcourse. Not every day and not very fast, but at least he was getting out. Now, however, he was getting lost and would wander across the grass even though there was a well-defined path. If I wasn't with him, he would walk aimlessly into the woods or turn and walk in the opposite direction. He was usually quite disoriented.

One evening Ray brought a glass of juice up to bed and set it on the night table. In the middle of the night he got up, and when he came back to bed sat on the night table instead of the bed. The glass tipped and got the bed and his shorts wet. I changed the bed while Ray went to get a clean pair of shorts. He went into the attached dressing area and came out wearing a bright yellow polo shirt—only his legs were through the arms and he was holding the bottom of the shirt around his waist. It was "hysterically" pathetic. He looked so funny and was so serious. Later he commented, "Apparently you take this much more seriously than I do." I thought, "Thank God."

Ray's eating was very erratic. He had always liked fruit juices and continued to drink them. But he ate very little. Though he was gradually losing weight, he continued to look well. He would often say that he wasn't hungry and sometimes ate no more than three to four hundred calories in a day.

Sometimes when Ray was unable to perform a task, we found that it would help to start him so as to trigger or jog his memory. It was kind of like revving up a motor. Once we got him started, he could often continue without—or at least with less—assistance. For example, when he didn't know how to pick up a sandwich on his plate, handing it to him, or actually putting it in his hand, seemed to trigger the memory of what to do, and then he could often eat by himself.

I began to think about options. I had already learned in my life that fantasizing possible scenarios was a way of preparing for them when, and if, they happened. I realized that I would not be able to handle what I knew to be an inevitability without preparing for it.

Our home was large enough that perhaps I could rent out the downstairs floor. It had a large family room with a fireplace, built-in floor-to-ceiling bookshelves, a built-in desk, and a separate entrance that led to a patio at the back of the house. It had a small bedroom and a bath. In addition, it had a large laundry room that could easily be used for a kitchen. It already had two sinks, cupboards, a plastic laminated counter, and a tile floor. Perhaps if I could rent the downstairs to a college student, it would pay for the cost of hiring someone to care for Ray. I would keep that option in mind. It might be possible also to find someone who would trade living downstairs for time spent with Ray.

There were services available in the city, but none that would meet our specific needs. Under a chore-workers program, people would come into a home for a few hours a day and do some housekeeping, make lunch, and attend to specific needs. But the waiting list was long, and the program did not provide the continual service we needed.

There were also nursing services that provided care for eight-hour shifts, but the cost of $40.00 a day took too large of a chunk from our income. Besides, Ray didn't need skilled nursing care. He needed a responsible person who would be sensitive to his needs and respect his dignity. We had no insurance coverage for "custodial care" at home or in a nursing home, should it become necessary to place Ray in one. Ray would be eligible for Medicare in two years, but that would not pay for nursing home care. How did families manage? Twenty to thirty thousand dollars a year. How could I possibly pay out that much and educate two children?

April 11

It has only been six or seven months since Ray was driving, dressing, and eating alone. He has deteriorated so quickly and it seems that there is nothing to be done. Part of me tells myself to accept what is happening. If Ray is deteriorating and losing his mental functioning without any hope for improvement, then let it happen quickly. I feel that I am losing him drip by drip; a kind of slow torture.

Ray's sleeping habits had changed drastically. He had always been a night person, reading well into the morning, and given the opportunity he liked to sleep in late. But now he was confused about night and day. He was often up all night, wandering around the house, unable to read or even watch TV. He seemed to have lost a sense of night and day. We tried tryptophan, a natural relaxant found in milk and often used for sleep disturbances. But it didn't help. I was reluctant to ask for a prescription for sleeping pills or a tranquilizer. I remembered the zombie-like state Ray had been in during the hospitalization.

With his endless wandering at night, I slept in snatches, getting up when I would hear Ray or reach over and not find him there. Even then there were times that I slept during near-catastrophes. I was always afraid that I would wake to find our house on fire, or Ray lying hurt somewhere.

Ray continued to slip. By the end of April, he was unable to select a pair of pants and a shirt from his closet, much less dress himself.

I couldn't discuss anything with him anymore. I continued to try to talk and plan with him, but it was of no use. At best he would lose the gist of a conversation after two or three sentences. His comprehension and thoughts seemed to come to a void, and then there was nothing. Although his vocabulary, grammar, and sentence structure remained relatively intact, what he said made little or no sense. He was losing the ability to link thoughts, to reason, to think. Sometimes I would open up to him about my pain. I had always turned to him, and he could always make me feel better. I continued to try, hoping to stir some feeling, some of the Ray I knew and needed. But he was oblivious. I would cry and he would just watch me, totally confused and probably somewhat threatened. He would not reach out; I would feel abandoned. He was there, and yet that iron-mesh screen prevented him from touching me.

We were walking at the parcourse one afternoon when I noticed that Ray had shaved. But as I looked closer I could see that he had only shaved half of his face. He looked so ridiculous. When we got home I tried to get him to shave the other side of his face, but he wouldn't. David brought the electric shaver to him and also tried to persuade him to finish shaving. But Ray refused. He said it hurt him. In fact, he got so upset over the whole incident that he said he would throw the shaver out of the window and me after it. The tears came. This was not the Ray I knew. I understood that he was confused. I knew that his responses stemmed from the progressive nature of a brain disorder, but I just couldn't seem to let it wash over me. It didn't seem to change how devastated I felt.

The next day I insisted that Ray had to shave before we could go to the parcourse. I just couldn't bear for someone to see him looking so absurd. He tried, but kept turning the shaver on and off, staring at it as if he were afraid of it. "It takes pieces out of me," he said. He would put the shaver to his face and then pull it away. We never did go to the parcourse that day.

Through the Alzheimer's support group I learned about *The 36-Hour Day* by Nancy L. Mace and Peter V. Rabins, a family guide for caregivers of persons with Alzheimer's disease and related dementing illnesses. It was clear to me how apt the title was, for I was finding that I needed to be alert and ready all the time. I would never know when Ray might need help or supervision of some kind. Rendering continuous care was becoming physically and emotionally exhausting.

I could not truly understand or accept what was happening. Before my very eyes I was losing Ray. We had not even said goodbye. He was with me physically, and yet he was not there at all. If he had had cancer or some slow, physically destructive disease that did not affect his brain, we would have talked and prepared. We would have said goodbye. I would wake from this nightmare one day and tell him what had happened. "You will not believe this incredible story, Honey," I would begin. Then I would recount the bizarre things that had happened. I would describe the feelings, the loss, the fear, the anger. He would reach out to me and take me in his arms, and I would feel his strength and be comforted. He would acknowledge how hard he knew it must have been for me and how proud he was. But it would be over. Now we could go ahead with our lives. It would be better than ever, for we would know what tragedy we were spared. We would value more than ever our time and life together. We would relish our ability to share, love, and enjoy each other. If only I could indeed awake from this living nightmare. If only!

SEVEN

I kept hoping for some improvement until the night in April when I talked to my friend Lily on the telephone. Lily had been my student teacher and then co-teacher when I was at the Ives School in Connecticut. She was thirteen years younger than I, but despite the age difference, we had become close friends; we could express to each other some of our deepest feelings.

Through Lily, Ray and I met Rich and watched him change from a gentle boyfriend into a husband and father of three. Rich was especially fond of Ray. Ray was a combination of the brother Rich never had and the father with whom he wanted to establish a closer relationship.

Rich later remembered those early days of their friendship: "I never knew a man who was so openly affectionate and loving with his sons. He taught me that masculinity need not be threatened by giving and nurturing. He taught me that it is okay to be free with touching and praise. It was just amazing to watch how much his kids loved him. The relationship was not like any father and son relationship I'd ever seen or experienced. The quality and time that Ray saved for his family was given without hesitation. It was how he expected it to be. I remember watching the interactions and hoping that somehow my relationship with my family could approach the openness and unity that Ray and Myrna and Michael and David shared. It was so very special. I loved Ray. I loved watching him love Myrna. Together they were certainly one."

I wanted to talk to Lily alone. But more and more often when I made a phone call, Ray would come and sit beside me. He seemed to shadow me in order to gain a sense of security. Sometimes he would just come to where I was and stand there, for what seemed to be no apparent reason. It must have made him feel safer.

So when I called Lily, Ray got on the phone too, as did Rich. As Ray talked, he was able to present himself as much less impaired than he actually was. He could mask his problems by speaking in generalities or by giving vague responses. Rich and Lily listened to Ray on the phone. He seemed normal, understandable, reasonable. But I was describing a different Ray. The two pictures were mutually exclusive.

Lily told me I needed to be more aggressive. "Myrna," she argued, "you can't just sit by and accept what they're telling you. You've got to demand more from the doctors. You've got to search for an answer." The more she talked, the worse I felt. I had called her for reassurance. I didn't know what else to do. I had done more than she seemed to realize. But I felt guilty. Maybe she was right; maybe I hadn't done enough.

Finally, I could stand it no longer. I became hysterical and screamed, "He's dying! I'm watching him die right in front of my eyes!" I hung up, ashamed. I shouldn't have said what I did in front of Ray, even though I knew it would not have an impact.

Ray was disturbed by my outburst, but not for the reason I would have expected. He did not respond to what I had said, or even to what Lily had said. Instead he told me, "How could you treat people like that? I don't know if I can ever forgive you." All I can surmise from the event was that Ray knew we were upset and had responded to my outbursts—my tone, not my words.

The Ray I knew would have taken me in his arms. He probably would have told me that I had overreacted, but would have mostly been concerned about how distraught I was feeling.

David heard what was going on and came to console me. Later, David told me that he thought I was so upset that I would kill myself. I assured him that I would never do that to him and Daddy. I explained that my outbursts of anger and despair were often cries for help but did not mean that I was about to give up the fight. There was no reason for him to be afraid, but I welcomed his strength when I did sink.

Lily called back later that evening. Rich had criticized her for being insensitive. I understood what Lily was feeling. I, too, felt that way sometimes. She couldn't accept the situation and wanted me to fight for a diagnosis that was treatable. But I didn't know what else to do. Who was I to see? Where was I to go? I didn't know the experts in the field—I wasn't even sure what field we were talking about. Neurology? Psychiatry?

But my conversation with Lily got the juices flowing again. I had become so wrapped up in the daily problems of Ray's failing memory that I had barely enough energy to make plans and expand my focus.

I telephoned a doctor at Massachusetts General Hospital who had written an article on normal pressure hydrocephalus. I called Dr. Weise and asked to see him. I wanted him to help plan the next step. I wrote a letter to some researchers at the Bronx VA Hospital, who referred me to another source. And I went back to the library.

For about one week in April of 1983 I seemed to feel there was some improvement. Ray opened a can of frozen lemonade, put the contents in a container, and added the proper amount of water. He helped with dinner one evening by taking fish out of a package and putting it in a baking dish. He turned on the correct burners on the stove three or four times, but had trouble turning them off. He seemed generally more alert and active. But there were still many problems.

I met with Dr. Weise, who—almost alone among the professionals we had consulted—offered counsel and support I'd come to depend on. I asked about seeking another opinion elsewhere. Although somewhat torn between his allegiance to his affiliated hospital and staff and what he honestly felt, he encouraged me to do so.

Before I left I told Dr. Weise about my ever-present feelings of loneliness and my pain at Ray's inability to appreciate or support me. I told him that even though I knew it was not in Ray's power to give me what I needed, I didn't know how to fill the void. So I continued to return to Ray and beg him to give me something he couldn't. Dr. Weise seemed to genuinely understand. That helped.

Ever since Ray had had the shunt surgery he had complained periodically of stomach pains. He described them as sharp, and I could tell he was in agony. I finally decided to call our family doctor. I was able to make the appointment at school, and the receptionist said the doctor could see Ray that morning. I tried to call Ray at home but got no answer. I left school; when I got home, Ray was asleep. I woke him, but he was angry and didn't want to get up. I begged Ray to get up. He just couldn't make any sense out of what I wanted him to do; all he wanted to do was stay in bed. I cried until he got up, but he refused to wash or shave. We got into the car, and I commiserated with myself about how difficult life was becoming.

In the doctor's office Ray was unable to follow the nurse's instructions. He did not understand that she wanted him to push up his sleeves so that she could take his blood pressure. He was unable to tell the doctor how long his stomach problem had existed. The doctor examined Ray, but found nothing. He said that he would contact the neurosurgeon to see if the problem might be neurologically based.

One rainy afternoon not long afterward, Ray and I started out to do some errands. He complained about the rain, remarking on how "terrible" it was. He was visibly disturbed by the weather and unable to handle the fact that it was raining.

In the car Ray said nothing. The silence between us was growing more apparent daily. There is a difference between a quiet, peaceful silence when two people know what is between them and the silence that now rose like a mountain between us. As much as I longed to move that mountain, I couldn't. But I couldn't accept it either.

I started to talk, knowing that I would be in agony when there was either no response or some disconnected, emotionless, nonsensical rejoinder. I had continued to look to Ray for something he could no longer provide. And Ray, helpless to change, could not comprehend my pain or the frightening changes within him.

I became so upset that I was unable to concentrate on the chores we planned to do. We came home. David asked why we had come back and Ray said, "Mommy and I had a fight." We did not fight. When people argue and disagree, it is a given that it is potentially possible for the conflict or problem to be resolved. At the very least, each party can understand the other's point of view. But we couldn't fight.

I went upstairs and lay on the bed and cried. Ray couldn't help what was happening, and there was nothing I could do to remedy it. I was losing Ray. I had really lost him already. All there was to do was cry.

In our life together Ray had always been totally accepting of me. He respected me and encouraged me to be myself. I needed to do that for him now: to love and accept him the way he was. I had to stop hurting him and myself by trying to bring back someone who was no longer there. I had to stop trying to change him back. I couldn't.

When I came downstairs, David told Ray to give me a hug. Ray walked over to me and stroked my head. His hands felt strong, but gentle. I closed my eyes remembering what was, savoring the caress, the tenderness and warmth that flowed through me, not knowing how much longer I would have even that. As he stroked me, he said he didn't know if I would want him to do that. I looked up at him and said, "That's all I want, Honey." The tears rolled down my cheeks and the ache spread through me.

April 24

About 1:30 this morning I smelled something. I did not jump out of bed as usual, but seemed to wake up slowly. When I got to the kitchen it was a mess. Ray had tried to make hot chocolate. He had put the chocolate and milk in a pot and then turned on two burners. Milk had boiled over, charred the pot, and the stove was filled with burned milk. He had put the pot in the sink, but let the water overflow so that it was all over the floor. He had used the paper toweling to try and clean the floor, but it was a river. One burner was still on. I realized how lucky it was that the paper towels did not come into contact with the burner. After I cleaned up, I told Ray that I thought we should think about having someone live with us to avoid problems like this. He seemed to understand.

When we went back to bed Ray told me that our bed was heavier in some places than in others. He didn't know why and I didn't understand what he meant.

I went to my second Alzheimer's support group meeting. The speaker was Marjorie Leigh, a family practitioner who specialized in gerontology. She explained what was understood about Alzheimer's disease: its insidious onset and the gradual and progressive course of the disease. She illustrated with a felt marker and a large flip pad the neurofibrillary tangles and plaques about which I had been hearing and reading. She compared Alzheimer's disease to multi-infarct dementia (MID).

Multi-infarct dementia, she explained, is associated with strokes and the presence of cardiovascular arteriosclerosis—a condition in which the walls of the arteries become thickened with fatty deposits, narrowing the flow of blood. Pathologically, the two types of dementia are quite different, although their effects can be quite similar.

Dr. Leigh seemed quite knowledgeable and patiently explained some very complicated neuropathology to a group of lay family members. As I had at the first meeting, I felt a community among these people. The questions, the nods of acknowledgment and familiarity when others shared their stories, the pain I saw on their faces and heard in their voices when they spoke of their personal plights, made me realize that each of them understood my pain, my loss, my grief.

After the meeting I stayed to talk with Marjorie. She was a lovely woman—petite, in her mid-to-late thirties, with straight, short black hair and an olive complexion. She listened sympathetically to the family members and seemed to understand their confusion. There was something I sensed in her from the beginning that was different.

The more I told Marjorie of Ray's history, the more intrigued she became. She asked questions and I eagerly poured forth the information. We walked out into the night air together, and I told her as much as I could in the short time we had.

She was particularly interested because Ray had just turned forty-seven. She was surprised that a brain biopsy had not been done at the time the shunt was inserted. I had asked Dr. Daniels about that at the time of the surgery, but had been told that it was usually not done any longer because frequently the biopsy findings did not reveal enough information to warrant the risk.

Marjorie felt, as Mark Weise and I did, that we needed to look elsewhere—perhaps a medical center that specialized in diseases causing dementia. There were a number of such places where specialists were doing research in the area of Alzheimer's disease and related disorders.

Before we left for the evening Marjorie took Ray's name and our telephone number, and asked if I would mind if she read Ray's hospital records. She would be in touch with me. I went home in ecstasy—partly because someone would help me and partly because I had just made a new friend.

Ray was still staying at home alone, and even though I called each day, I knew that he was not able to handle the situations that arose. One day Ray said someone had called. He said it had something to do with Dr. Cameron, our family physician, but he couldn't tell me any more than that. I asked him who had talked the most, trying to ascertain whether the caller was giving or trying to obtain information. He said that he had done more of the talking, which made me think that whoever had called had asked him something. But, when I asked what he had talked about, he couldn't remember. I didn't know if someone was trying to change the appointment we had for the following week or what.

Sometimes Ray would remember that someone had called, but could hardly ever remember the message or conversation. One day he tried to take a telephone message from Michael. He had written something and I could make out a little of the scrawl, but was unable to understand its meaning.

April 28

Ray went out to get the mail twice today even though I had told him that it had come already. Later in the afternoon, when I was tutoring Jamie (a youngster that I saw once a week) he came into the kitchen. We were studying state capitals. There was a time when Ray knew all the state capitals. In fact, there were games we would play with the kids on automobile trips with the states and their capitals. I asked Ray if he thought he remembered the capitals. He said he thought he did. We asked him some and he was able to give a few, but was completely blank on others. Jamie, the youngster I was tutoring, asked Ray the capital of Nebraska and he said he didn't know. When Jamie said it was Lincoln, Ray asked, "Is that the state?"

Ray and I continued to go to the parcourse, but less frequently. By the time I got home from school and got him ready, it was usually growing dark. One afternoon when we got there, Ray was very disoriented and had great difficulty getting out of the car. He did not seem to know where he was supposed to go, and I literally had to pull him along a clearly designated path. He kept asking, "Is this right?" At one point he made a face as if to say, "What's with me? Why can't I do this?"

It was late by the time we arrived and beginning to grow dark. It was warm and the fragrances of the early spring changes brought back nostalgic reminders of the summer camp where Ray and I had met and fallen in love. The memories loomed vividly in my mind, and the surrounding smells were so pronounced that the bittersweet feelings became almost unbearable. I held on to Ray's hand, now as much to guide him as to be close. His hair was beginning to grow back since the surgery, and he looked much as he did when I had first met him and he had had a crewcut. I put my arm around him as we walked, and he responded by putting his arm around me. But I know he did not remember as I did. I cried and he responded with a smile and a gentle laugh—the kind of laugh I remembered when he was touched by my reaction to something.

It was strange, but in spite of the pain of surfacing memories, there was an element of pleasantness. At least Ray was there. I could touch him and for those precious minutes pretend he was my old honey.

Our twenty-third wedding anniversary was April 30, and it brought memories of other occasions. With mixed pleasure and pain, I found myself remembering our seventeenth wedding anniversary, which we had spent in Stockbridge, Massachusetts. The weather was perfect April-May weather and it had been a particularly romantic, tender, and close time for both of us. We walked the streets of the small, historic city, drove through the countryside, and visited the Norman Rockwell Museum.

We had a wonderful lunch at a small restaurant. For some reason we began to reminisce about our years together, sharing memories of our meeting at camp; living in New York; the births of our children; jobs; friends; funny, difficult, and warm times. Ray would remind me of a particular time he remembered and I would recall something that perhaps he had forgotten. We laughed and interrupted each other as we eagerly exchanged memories. It was clear to both of us what we had and needed to hold on to. We held hands across the table. Ray squeezed my hand and just smiled. I knew what the smile and the squeeze meant. I loved him so very much. He was a treasure with which I could never part.

We stayed at the Red Lion Inn in the heart of the city—an old quaint inn with a balcony. Below our room was the dining room where we had dinner. The piano that had been background dinner music could be heard in our room. But with a chill, I now remembered the next morning: Ray awoke unable to speak. He could make sounds, but not formulate words. It lasted for about ten minutes and then passed. That had been six years before.

On April 30, 1960, we had been married by a justice of the peace in Yonkers, New York. We had planned to be married in Detroit where my parents lived and I grew up. But I had been living and going to school in New York. My mother would have had to plan the wedding since I was so far away. Besides, Ray's mother, Sarah, had already found us an apartment. And August seemed a long time away. For us it really didn't matter much. We were together.

I had been staying with Ray's parents in Brighton Beach. Knowing the superintendent and being the highest bidder could land an eager renter an apartment in a rent-controlled building in 1960. And Sarah was a master of the art. She found us a one-room apartment in a prewar six-floor building.

Ray's family lived in a two-bedroom apartment, which was home for Ray's parents and three children. My presence, although welcomed, made the quarters that much more cramped. So it was to Sarah's advantage that I move into "our" apartment to await the wedding. My parents, eager not to be grandparents prior to nine months of wedded bliss, encouraged us to marry before our August plans. And so we had.

One Saturday, after being given blood tests by a neighborhood doctor who was a friend of the family's (he told Sarah that he didn't give the marriage six months), we drove to Yonkers. We had planned to be married in the city, but were unable to because I was under twenty-one. Warren, Ray's best friend, and his parents went. Goldie, Warren's wife, had the measles.

We stopped at the Cross County Shopping Center Mall, checked the phone book, and called a justice of the peace who invited us to come over. We were greeted at the door by the judge's wife, who ushered us into his study, where he sat, one leg up on his desk, because he suffered from gout. I wore a plain navy blue dress and only remember feeling that the whole thing seemed anticlimatic. We were married, but nothing was really different. I guess I just felt as if we had legalized that which had already taken place. We needed no one to tell us what commitment meant. I think we knew that even then. We truly wanted to be united and together. I don't remember having any doubts. Maybe I was too naive, too much of a romantic. But I believed at age twenty that I would live happily ever after with this man who really was still very much of a boy.

We had our wedding breakfast at the Howard Johnson's near

the shopping center where we had stopped to call the justice of the peace, and then headed home. We dropped Warren and Ray's parents off and then went to Waldbaum's for some groceries. Ray had to be back at work and I had school on Monday.

In Waldbaum's we pushed our shopping cart, both aware of the brand-new bands on our left hands. I was sure that everyone in the store knew that we were newlyweds. I felt as if I were wearing a neon sign. In the store we bumped into a friend of Ray's whom he had not seen in a long time. They greeted each other, and then the other fellow introduced his new wife to us. Ray introduced me as his wife, and the fellow looked surprised and said, "I didn't know that you were married. When were you married?" Ray answered, "This morning." And the fellow quipped, "What the hell are you doing here?" That was our first wedding.

In August, four months later, my parents came to New York. My father brought my grandmother's gold wedding band. Although Ray and I were married, we knew that it was important to my parents that we have a religious ceremony. One day shortly before they were to leave, we spent the afternoon in Coney Island, and returned home dressed in shorts and sneakers. Across the street from my in-laws' apartment house, my parents saw a sign in a first-floor apartment window: RABBI ABRAHAM DORTMAN—MARRIAGES PERFORMED.

The rabbi invited us in and Ray told him we would like to be married tomorrow. I do not remember why the rabbi said that this was not possible, but do remember quite clearly how concerned he was about our urgency. Now, twenty-four years later, I can still remember his exact words spoken with a Yiddish accent, "Why are you in such a hurry? You can tell me. I'm like a *doctor*." Ray assured him that the only reason we were anxious to have the service performed so soon was because my parents were leaving. Reluctantly, he agreed to marry us on the spot.

Ray went across the street to summon his parents. Since the rabbi was an orthodox rabbi, the women, as well as the men, would have to cover their heads. My mother found some plastic rain hats in her purse for the occasion, which she proudly handed Sarah and me. The rabbi provided the yarmulkes, as well as a witness, a man who happened to be outside the apartment building. Ray knew the witness—an old man in the neighborhood, name unknown, who used to chase the kids from wherever they seemed to be playing. He did not recognize Ray.

The rabbi brought out a canopy to hold over us during the ceremony. Our parents each held a pole. The rabbi began to chant the service. He must have been a stroke victim, because he had great difficulty controlling the saliva in his mouth and literally spit his words at us.

At one point during the ceremony the rabbi turned to fill a wine glass from which we were to drink. Ray leaned over to kiss me. My father, thinking that we thought the service was over, walked toward us holding his pole to tell us, "Not yet." As he came to us, the canopy collapsed. The rabbi turned to hand us the wine and found the canopy on our heads. We quickly repositioned ourselves for the rest of the ceremony and ended with Ray breaking the traditional glass for good luck. The rabbi's wife served her guests the Ritz crackers she had in the house. Mazel tov!

Now it was our twenty-third anniversary. I did some yard work late that afternoon and jealously watched some of our neighbors leave to go out on this Saturday evening. I was really indulging in self-pity and thought about my life, my life with the Ray I had known. I knew I would never laugh with Ray again. We would never enjoy each other as we had again. I felt cheated and angry.

That evening neighbors asked us to go out with them for ice cream. Ray hardly uttered a word the entire evening. He was very confused about how to get in and out of the car. He often forgot how to put one leg in first in order to sit down. He would just stand by the car door completely blank about what to do. Sometimes I would have to pick his leg up to trigger the memory. Sometimes the memory would come back by itself. Sometimes it didn't. When he got out of the car, the same kind of thing happened. He just sat there, not knowing how to begin. Sometimes a verbal reminder was sufficient; sometimes a tug on the arm brought back the process. Other times my moving one of his legs—and sometimes both—and pulling his arms was the only thing that worked. There was no consistency.

In the restaurant Ray did not remember what he liked so I chose and ordered his favorite all-chocolate ice-cream soda for him. Ray said nothing during the forty-five minutes the four of us sat together; he seemed content, though, and was able to eat the ice cream without help. When the check came, I handled the money. It was like taking a small child out. The tears that came forth in bed that night confused Ray as much as ever.

May 2

I recorded part of a conversation Ray and I had today. How aware he must be of his confusion and fear at times!

RAY: You're [talking to me] like a smurf, no texture. It's like you're liquid, just flow, don't resist. It's hard to explain. Everything's fragmented, falling apart. I don't know what I mean. I did know, but I don't know now.

ME: You sound angry. Are you angry with me?

RAY: I get a feeling of being blamed. If only I could control myself, my destiny, my fate. Somehow I'm responsible. You look to me for so much more. It's not there.

May 4

Ray put his shirt and sweater on backwards today. When I pointed it out to him he was confused as to what to do about it. I had to help him take it off and put it on the right way. He kept asking, "Is this right?" He frequently asks me if he's all dressed. He's never sure if he's finished, if he's put on everything he's supposed to.

Ray went for abdominal X-rays and a sonogram today to determine why he's been having pains in his abdomen. In the office I had to go back and help him dress and undress. I know the technicians didn't know what was the matter, but I find I'm getting more used to helping Ray without feeling I owe some kind of an explanation to anyone. He's so helpless and dependent on me that I have to block out feelings of embarrassment.

About a week after the Alzheimer's meeting, Marjorie, the family practitioner, called and asked if she and her fiancé, Stuart, a psychologist, could come over and meet Ray. It was her vacation, and she wanted to see Ray in his own environment. She had read all the records that were available at the hospital. I was terribly excited.

Marjorie and Stuart spent about an hour and a half with us. I made myself keep quiet, not answering or correcting so that Marjorie could learn what she could from Ray himself. As usual, he was able to present a much better picture of himself than I knew to be the case. Somehow Ray's social skills remained sufficiently intact. But, in spite of the facade, Marjorie was able to see some of the problems.

She asked Ray a lot of questions about specific problems he was having, what his concerns were, what he thought about work, how long ago all this might have begun. He had a lot of difficulty remembering things, and although initially he acted relatively alert, he was unable to conceal his memory loss when asked specific questions.

Marjorie's comment when she left that afternoon was that she felt that Ray's problem was primarily dementia and that its onset was a long time ago, getting progressively worse in the last months. She told me that she had called our house right after the last Alzheimer's meeting. She needed Ray's first name and date of birth to get his records. He was able to give her both pieces of information but had not remembered to tell me. Could that have been the time he told me Dr. Cameron's office had called? I never had been able to track down the call. I wondered.

A few days after Marjorie's visit, she called to tell me that she had contacted Dr. Abraham Hindle, a neurologist at Duke University Medical Center. I knew of Dr. Hindle and had even had an occasion to speak with him on the phone. He was a key person in the field of Alzheimer's disease, and Duke was doing important research in Alzheimer's and related disorders.

Marjorie said that Dr. Hindle was interested in taking the case. My job was to round up all the records that were not available to her: Ray's CAT scan and report from a year earlier, when Ray first experienced numbness; records from our family physician; and records from Ray's recent kidney diagnosis. She would make the arrangements.

May 7

At night, in bed especially, the pain and enormity of it all hits. Sometimes I beg God to let me have Ray again just for a while. Just to help make some decisions, just to share some final words of love and commitment. Knowing that I have lost him is a pain, I think, no worse than if he died.

May 8

Ray woke this morning and asked for coffee. He wandered around the house looking for something. He couldn't think of what he wanted. He said, "It is just like juice—interchangeable with juice, but not juice." I named other liquids, but was not able to identify the one (if any) he was thinking of. He continued to wander around the house. Then he spotted a notebook in my school bag. "Could you get thinner ones?" He asked. "I don't know if you could find them," he added. His speech was slow and he had great difficulty expressing himself. "Pay no attention to me," he said. "You can't even answer me, can you?"

"No, I can't, Honey. I want to, but I can't."

Ray is having more trouble with verbal expression, more difficulty retrieving specific words. He often tries, but then gives up trying to express an idea because it becomes too difficult and frustrating for him. He seems to know what he wants to say, but can't put it all together.

Ray came out to watch while I was working in the yard this

afternoon. At one point I realized that our Mazda was parked in the middle, rather than at the top, of the driveway. I commented about it and Ray said that he had moved it. When I asked why, he said, "My leg hurt and I had to change gears."

May 12

Last night Ray's left arm went numb for about ten minutes. He wasn't sure, said he thought it was numb. When he woke at night, he had to go to the bathroom, but didn't know where it was. I walked him to the bathroom, but he did not remember how to urinate. I had to tell him exactly what to do. But the verbal prompts did not help much. I could see that he was experiencing some urgency, but did not know how to proceed. Although he resisted, seeming to realize that it was somehow degrading, it was necessary for me to physically help him through the steps.

At dinner last night Ray didn't know how to begin to eat. Michael, home for the summer, told him to pick up the hamburger from his plate. He looked confused, but once he took it in his hands, was able to continue. There are more and more occasions when he needs help.

Ray was watching TV this evening when he became aware of his confused state. Usually, he just sits there and I can't tell how much he is absorbing. But tonight they ran a series of thirty-second commercials. Ray just couldn't keep up with the changes. He did not have the time or ability to process what was happening and he knew it. I could tell by his sighs of frustration and his shifting uncomfortably in his chair. But his only comment was, "Don't know what these guys are doing." He did not have the insight or words to convey the loss.

EIGHT

In the middle of May, Ray went for a third battery of tests. The examiner said that there was a noticeable change in Ray. When she had first tested him, he did not seem abnormal until she actually began the testing. But now it was apparent, just speaking with him, that there was considerable deterioration. Part of this, she felt, was because of his hair, still struggling to achieve a bit more than a crewcut. But, in addition, there was a vagueness and confusion about him that anyone would notice at first.

After the testing Ray stayed in the waiting room while I spoke with Dr. Weise. I asked Ray whether he minded if I saw Mark alone. He said that he didn't, and even when I came out of Mark's office, he did not seem concerned about what may have been discussed.

Mark started by saying that the previous testing had remained fairly stable. "This time," he went on, "there has been a dramatic decline." Ray's verbal IQ was now eighty-four; his performance IQ was fifty-seven; and he had an overall score of seventy-one. There was about a twenty-point loss in a matter of four months.

I was prepared for those findings, but not for the rest. Mark showed me three drawings Ray had done. First, he was asked to copy a model. Then he was asked to do the same drawing without a model from which to copy, and, after a delayed period of time, was again asked to reproduce the drawing. As I looked at the drawings I felt a stabbing, piercing pain in my chest. I couldn't believe what I was looking at I visualized a split image: On one side were the precise, professional elevations, perspectives, clever nebbishes, and architectural printing that Ray

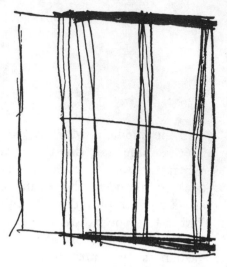

Asked to remember and redraw
a complex figure in May 1983,
Ray produced this crude sketch.

After a delay, doctors asked
him to redraw the figure again.

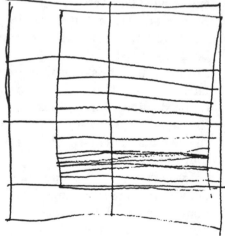

Curiously, Ray produced the crudest
drawing while looking directly at the
original.

had always done so skillfully. On the other side were the scrawls of a child, maybe a three- or four-year-old. I was devastated. I knew that Ray had been in agony when he was in that room trying to draw. I knew that he knew that he was doing poorly. In fact, when he came out from the testing, before I saw Mark, he had been visibly depressed. He didn't say anything, but when I asked him if the tests were hard, he said, "Yes." This man whose kids thought he was the smartest person in the world, who delighted in reading, who could recite lines of his favorite movies, who was so gifted and talented, who wrote as well as he spoke, who was a master at trivia—this man now acknowledged that tasks that children could perform were too hard for him.

Mark was shocked by the accelerated decline. He doubted that Ray had Alzheimer's disease. The new CAT scans did not indicate any shrinking or atrophy of the brain; besides, the deterioration was unusually rapid for Alzheimer's disease. "But," he told me, "if he keeps this acceleration up, he will be a total invalid with no self-care skills by the end of the summer."

We talked about care for Ray. Mark told me quite candidly that I should not be looking for someone to live with us who would watch Ray on the side. Ray would need much more care than that. I had one more month of school, but I knew that after the summer I could no longer put off getting help for Ray. I was not surprised by what Mark said, but hearing it made it more real—and harder.

I told Mark about Marjorie Leigh's interest in Ray's case and the fact that I was planning to go to Duke with Ray. Although Mark had concurred with my need to get a second opinion, he now questioned the value of such a move. But I knew I was not satisfied with what had been done so far. No one really was following Ray's case. The neurosurgeon had placed the shunt and would see Ray every few months to make sure it was functioning. But that wasn't the problem. He was deteriorating weekly, and I still wasn't sure they really knew what was wrong with him. I had to find out.

In the car going home, I told Ray that Mark had said there had been a slight loss. He said, "Really?" and seemed surprised. Although he had moments of intense awareness, most of the time Ray seemed oblivious to his condition. It was the only merciful aspect of the disease that was relentlessly destroying him.

May 13

At school this morning Clay, my devil-may-care, hyperactive third-grader came in. He was very sad and said his dad, who was laid-off from work, would only get unemployment for another week. Then they wouldn't have any money. I made some banal remark like, "Everything will work out okay." Then I told him to come and let me hug him. He came over and I held him on my lap awhile. He put his head on my shoulder and we just sat there. Neither of us said anything. The tears fell. I guess they were for all the sadness around. In a way Clay's fears are no less than mine. I am learning that pain, hurt, fear are not qualitative.

May 14

Out of the blue Ray asked, "When are we going?" We had not talked about doing anything in the afternoon. I asked where? To cover the fact that he did not know, he answered, "To the activity of the day."

At dinner tonight Ray asked for the mustard. It was in front of him, but he asked, "Where is the balance of mustard?" His choice of vocabulary, as well as content, often seems inappropriate lately. In attempting to put butter on a potato, he cut a piece of butter, but could not pick it up. He made a number of futile attempts, sometimes spearing a piece with a fork, but then placing it on top of the butter from which he had cut it. Finally I helped him.

May 15

I am feeling less and less hope lately and more and more the impact of losing Ray. I worry what will happen to me. He provided so much emotional security that I have become a more confident and self-assured person. I am terrified to lose that.

Sometimes I fantasize my life after Ray. I guess I want to feel there will be another life for me. I find that I look at other men, think about qualities that I would want them to have, wonder what it would be like. Could I ever share and care for someone else, sleep with and love anyone again? Who would want me? I'm 43—not so old for an already established, loving relationship. But who's looking for a 43-year-old? I'm not always so sure that I'll make it or even want to. I'm not sure that, if it weren't for the kids, I wouldn't want to go peacefully with Ray.

May 17

I think Ray was up a lot last night. I had fallen asleep on the couch in the den. He woke me to go to bed about 11:30. As I walked through the den and the kitchen, I saw that there were four or five cigarettes on the table in the den, about ten slices of bread stacked on the kitchen table, and a shoe on the kitchen counter.

In the morning when I awoke, Ray was already dressed. He had on two pairs of pants and two shirts. He said that he had to get dressed. He said that he had wet his pants, but didn't know where. I didn't know if he really had, and was unable to find any evidence of a problem. Although he has been having some difficulty anticipating when he has to use the bathroom, as far as I know, he has managed.

Ray was rapidly deteriorating, and the lawyer I had contacted had not yet called us to come in and sign the documents that we had drawn. I called him to let him know that time was becoming a factor. I did not know how competent Ray would be if we waited much longer. We set up an appointment for the following week.

Ray responded to many questions with answers that demonstrated his attempts at coping with his loss of memory. His answers were often not germane to the subject. Instead, they seemed to be intrusive kinds of remarks, thoughts that were triggered by a single word or association. Listening to him, one was not sure how related his comments were. They often seemed to be on the periphery of making sense. When asked if he knew why I was upset, Ray once said, "I think it's a mental state—that you have relented." Or asked what he thought they would do at Duke? He said, "I guess I'll have to sign in."

He also had great difficulty retrieving information and would sometimes solicit help from us by giving us clues as to what he was attempting to recall. One day he was trying to remember the names of our friends Lily and Rich. But failing to recall their names, he asked, "Do you think I'll see my friends again? The boy and girl?"

Because his vocabulary and syntax masked his inability to reason, it was only after experiencing this pattern of response over a period of time that I was able to understand the extent to which Ray's memory and other cognitive functions were impaired.

In spite of Ray's confusion, disorientation, and general deterioration, some of his mental capacity was still intact. He was well aware of salvaged bits of memory and seemed pleased with himself when the boys and I marveled at what he had retained. Ray remembered many pieces of factual information and could give definitions of uncommon and even esoteric words, attesting to his once-extensive vocabulary. But these were islands of memory without connecting bridges—they were detached, isolated, fragmented.

The bathroom became a problem faster than I had anticipated. Sometimes Ray couldn't find the bathroom; and he soon was not able to anticipate when he had to urinate. By the time he did know, it was always with a sense of urgency. Although not consistently, Ray was becoming incontinent. I had two more weeks of school. The summer would mean that some major decision would have to be made

All was not doom and gloom, even though it often seemed that way. Ray's putting clothes on backwards, saying some of the nonsensical things he did, still joking about things he remembered, brought some laughter into our home. Often it was a choice of how to look at a situation. Sometimes it was emotionally easier to find the humor in it.

One afternoon when I got home from school, Ray told me that we were going away for the weekend. He said he had made plans to visit a place and to buy some property. Someone had called and offered us a free weekend at some resort, if we would tour the grounds and listen to a sales pitch. I couldn't help thinking how the conversation must have gone between Ray and the salesperson, and the thought made me chuckle a little. Later that evening someone called to confirm our weekend appointment. I canceled.

Ray became more and more disoriented in his own environment. He wandered every night. It was not unusual for him to have to use the bathroom three or four times during the night. We put a night light in the bathroom, hoping that would help orient him. It may have for a brief period, but after a while, it made no difference. Ray would wander from one room to another. His wandering often seemed aimless. At other times he initially appeared to have some direction and purpose, but would either forget or lose his way. Then, without a sense of where he was or what to do, he would relieve himself wherever he happened to be.

I became very sensitive to his getting up at night. I would walk him to the bathroom and stand him in front of the toilet. That was often sufficient. Ray would come back to bed and try to get in on my side, even though he had to walk around the bed to get to me. Even when he would see me lying there, he could not comprehend that he could not lie down there. Sometimes I thought he knew, as he did in other instances, that something wasn't right, but just didn't know what to do to rectify the problem. He was not able to understand the verbal instructions I would give him to go to his side. I would have to get out of bed, take his hand, and walk him around to the other side of the bed.

Even then there were many times that he did not know how to get into bed. He might sit at the foot of the bed, and when he tried to lie down would not be able to reach the head of the bed. There he would lie, his head in the middle of the bed, uncovered, and curled up in a fetal position. I would have to take his arms and help him up so we could try again. Sometimes he would forget how to even sit and lie down. I would have to physically prompt the motor pattern to get him started, or sometimes actually move him into a prone position. He would become very frustrated and seemed to know how dependent and helpless he was.

May 19

It's always at night that it hits me the hardest. I begin to give in to all of the trials of the day that I've put on a back burner so that I can function. But at night, in bed with Ray, I become so weak. I cried a long time last night and told Ray, in as many ways as I could, how much he means to me, how much I need him, and how special he has always been. He did not understand, but after a long time of my crying, he reached over and held me. There is still some instinct within him that surfaces occasionally that seems to recognize when I am troubled. Some-.times he reacts by being angry because it must be threatening and disturbing in some way to him. But there are those rare moments when he does reach out.

I felt the strength and protection that is now only a memory; I melted when he touched me. I felt safe and loved. He made love to me, and as he did, I found I was savoring it; telling myself to hold the feeling, remember for the time when it would be gone. It wasn't like lovemaking had been before for me, but rather some semblance of closeness and intimacy that I desperately tried to capture and hold, fearing it will never be again.

It was 3 A.M. when Ray woke me calling, "Help me." I found him in the bathroom standing in the dark. I don't know how long he had been calling for help, but he had become frightened when he realized he didn't know how to get out of the dark bathroom. He was upset and angry with himself.

By the end of May Ray was unable to shower or shave without assistance. We would have to put shampoo on his head, adjust the water, and turn it off. We were already laying out the clothes he was to wear for the day; he wore anything we put out. He had loved clothes and taken pride in keeping his wardrobe replenished and in good condition. His clothes were carefully chosen and well tailored. But now he often looked disheveled and unkempt. He frequently refused to shave, and by the time I would insist, ready to do battle, he would complain that it hurt, even though he used an electric shaver. When he did shave, he would move the shaver in one area over and over again. I'd move his hand to another part of his face, but he'd go back and shave an area that was already done.

On one occasion David and I spent forty minutes shaving Ray. We employed all of the skills, tricks, and distractions that we had learned over the last months and found the ordeal extremely draining. I remember that when we finished, we stood in the bathroom and shook hands, congratulating each other on a job maybe not well done but at least accomplished.

I dreaded the nights. Ray had lost his perception of day and night. He got up so frequently that I could only sleep an hour or two at a time. I was a good sleeper and found that I could fall back to sleep easily. But uninterrupted sleep became a thing of the past. Sometimes it got to me.

Around three o'clock one morning Ray woke me. He wanted me to make him some hot milk. We had decided that it might help him since the tryptophan did not, and I was still terribly reluctant to have him take any sleeping medications. I was concerned about damage to his kidneys, and also did not want to see him any more passive than he already was. I attempted to get him to try to sleep without the milk, dreading to have to get up again, but it was to no avail.

When I got out of bed, I found that for the first time I was mad and resentful at having to be at Ray's beck and call. I slammed the pot down on the stove and hit the wall with my fist. I heated the milk and brought it upstairs, putting it on the night table beside Ray. I was angry. It sure wasn't Ray's fault, but I was sick of giving and giving and getting nothing.

There were not many occasions like that, but they were

there. Moments when I wondered when it would be my turn. Times I wanted to run away.

May 23

I have no other life anymore. I dress Ray, help him shower and shave, help him find his way around the house, help him eat, watch him so that he doesn't do something dangerous. We don't even talk. Two people that could sit for hours and find fulfill-ment in that now spend hours in virtual silence. I am now a caregiver. I go to work and then come home to a man who de-pends on me to help him get through life at its most primitive level. I can not and will not turn my back on him, but I cannot endure the loneliness and emptiness that go with it. I scream out for help. But there is no one there to make it go away. I'm living a nightmare, and the night goes on.

May 24

Our appointment with the lawyer and the trust represen-tative from the bank was today. Michael and Ray met me at the bank. Michael had showered, shaved, and dressed Ray. He was so proud of himself and asked me a couple of times how Daddy looked. Ray was wearing a suit and tie and Michael lovingly held his hand, guiding him up the elevator and into the offices where we were to sign the documents.

The lawyer, bank representative, and a few secretaries were there to witness the signatures. The lawyer asked Ray some questions to ascertain his competency. First, he asked if Ray knew what a power of attorney was. I remember that Ray gave a very clear and articulate answer, in much the same way he could often do when we would ask him a definition of a word. The lawyer also asked him if he knew who I was, and if he trusted me to make decisions for him, should it become neces-sary. Again, he answered and did seem to understand why we were there. I signed the papers that the lawyer passed to me and then it was time for Ray to do the same. Ray found it almost impossible to remember how to sign his name. He was even un-able to place the pen on the correct line, let alone execute his signature. The attorney walked over to Ray, and standing behind his chair, placed Ray's hand on the line where he was to sign, while verbally telling him to make an R. Eventually, Ray's memory was jarred, but the result was a signature that barely represented one I recognized.

All the papers were signed, and although I felt a sense of relief, a wave of that sick feeling, which I knew to be grief, flooded my body. I don't think I have ever experienced such a feeling before.

As we sat in the bank conference room, I remembered how sharp and astute Ray would have been in this setting. We had always thought that he was a frustrated lawyer. He loved to argue an issue, knew legal jargon, which he often used when writing business letters, and had even rewritten a contract for a condominium we were to buy, which to his surprise, was accepted. Now he must have seemed like a lamentable soul. He sat in this room without a word, having been brought to this meeting by his nineteen-year-old son, without whom he would not have been able to wash, shave, dress, travel, or find his way.

I was so sorry that no one here had known Ray when he was well and wanted to tell them, "You should have known him before. You would not believe what has happened to this man. I wish you could have known him."

Life was becoming a series of what-nexts. One evening Ray was wandering around the house as he often did. He seemed aimless, even lost. I asked him what he was doing and he replied, "Wandering around in the dark." I was never able to determine how much, if any, humor Ray found in his situation. I believe that he was often semi-aware of his plight, and remarks such as this were said in both truth and jest.

He would ask the same questions over and over again because he had forgotten that he had just asked them. He would follow David and me around the house or call to see where we were. But since he often was so disoriented, unless he could see us, he became frightened and insecure. He would look for confirmation from us when he was confused and often ask, "Is that what I want?" Once he accused me of lying to him when I told him I had tried to buy some Nova Scotia salmon but was not able to find a store that had it in stock.

May 25

I went up to bed about 10 P.M. Ray came up, too, even though he had gotten up late today. About 11 P.M. I woke to find Ray voiding on the bedroom floor. I spent the next hour changing him into some clean clothing, cleaning the carpet, warming some milk, getting him into bed, and covering him with some extra blankets since he has been so cold at night lately. Then I cried.

One evening I asked Ray what was the happiest thing in his life. He said he was proud of his work. Then I asked him about special people in his life (obviously hoping he'd say me). First he said Eleanor—hated her, loved her. I asked him about the kids. He said he loved them unconditionally. Then I asked him about his love for me and waited eagerly for his reply. He said he had some reservations. My heart sank, and the hurt covered my very being. I knew he really didn't understand or mean what he said. Why did I set myself up like that? I knew why. I was so desperate for his love and affection that I took those kinds of chances. But I couldn't deal with the devastating effects. I had to learn to stop doing that to myself. I had to learn that what was lost was really gone, no longer a part of who he and I were.

When I told Ray why I was upset he answered by telling me he loved me. I told him I couldn't stand what was happening, and he said, "I'll be okay. We have to believe that we'll be okay."

Often I would write in my journal as Ray spoke so that I could get accurate quotes. When I asked him if he minded, he said, "No, at least you take me seriously."

Occasionally he would comment on something going on in the world. Ray had always been quite socially and politically aware. He had been strongly opposed to our involvement in Vietnam before it was fashionable; he had been a supporter of women's liberation and arms limitations; he had opposed Nixon, capital punishment, and Jesse Helms. He must have been very concerned about America's defense policies one day when he said, "I think we will be judged to be bad guys. This whole aid thing. Maybe I shouldn't be concerned. We're on the verge of momentous decisions. We're going to be held accountable."

Gradually, I had explained what was happening to people in our neighborhood. It was becoming painfully apparent that something was seriously wrong with Ray. He wasn't working, his head had been shaved, he needed help getting in and out of the car, he seemed disoriented. I knew of buzzing and concern among the neighbors and was aware they were hesitant to approach me and ask about the situation. But as things became clearer to me, I found I was able to, and even needed to, trust and share with others. I knew, too, that I would need to call on them in the event I needed help.

There were times when Ray wandered to different families' homes on our block. Sometimes I didn't know that he had wandered away, and it was both a support and a relief to know how sensitively others would talk to him, take his hand, and walk him home.

One Sunday afternoon Ray went into the bathroom and closed the door. But instead of opening the door to come out, he opened a drawer which prevented him from opening the door. He could not get out and I could not get in. He could not understand that he needed to close the drawer so that he could open the door. The boys were not home. I called the next-door neighbors, mostly to alert them that I might need their help. Somehow, after about a half hour, Ray's memory jarred long enough for him to close the drawer. The incident was over. But it was reassuring to know that there was help available, should I need it.

May 31
When you're really committed to someone, they come first in your life. Ray was committed to me and I to him. Nothing, in

the long run, mattered quite as much as each other. And now I have no one committed to me in that way. The kids are great. They have been there for both of us and I know I can depend on them. But they each must lead their own lives. They cannot and should not commit to me the way Ray did. My parents, friends . . . no one. It is only Ray whose life was so intertwined in mine that I knew he would always be there. We had an investment in each other. We knew we could always count on the other. Others may care, give me time, love me. But no one is there for me like he was. That realization is unbearable—perhaps selfish—but nevertheless, unbearable.

I found I was becoming interested in the lives of divorced and separated people I knew. In some ways I would identify with them. I wondered what would happen to me. I was so incredibly lonely and sad and didn't know how to "get on with my life." How was I to cope with this? How could I start to make the pain go away? Ray's presence, touch, sweetness, voice, smell—those were constant reminders of what was. A scene, a song, an expression, a word—twenty-three years of memories. How could I not feel? How could I protect myself and still stay mentally and emotionally healthy? I didn't know.

June 3

I think something new is beginning to happen that makes me very sad. I find that I am turning to Ray less. Instead of crying during the past few days, begging to have him return, I find I pull away. I get the juice, make dinner, do the things that have to be done, but in a custodial way, not with the love I felt before. This evening Ray asked me to go to the movies and I said that I didn't want to. The thought of going brought feelings of embarrassment and hard work. When I go somewhere with Ray it is going with someone for whom I am a caregiver. He is no longer my friend, husband, lover. My relationship with Ray is now totally caring for his physical needs and trying to provide a buffer to the outside world. I cannot share with him, go to him for emotional support, have fun with him. And I guess, even though he is not responsible for what has happened, that I feel angry with him. The thought of going to the beach, out to dinner, or anything social without him is still very difficult for me. I can't go with him, but it's hard to go without him. He is still aware enough of what's going on so that I feel guilty about my feelings. But I need to do some things for myself, too.

We seem to be in a state of limbo. I feel like I'm on a treadmill and can't get off. I have a husband, but not a husband. He is physically present and mentally alert enough for me to still consider him as a person who has feelings, thoughts, and is somewhat aware. But he does not provide anything for me. I don't know how to fill the void. I think I am protecting myself by feeling this rejection. I hope this feeling doesn't last long, but it certainly is less painful in some ways.

June 6

Ray wanted to make pork chops for dinner tonight. He took out Chinese sweet and sour sauce and seafood cocktail sauce. There was a glass of pineapple-grapefruit juice on the counter. He wanted to make a sauce by mixing the three ingredients. I thought it was a strange concoction, but Ray insisted that it was okay. So I mixed the three ingredients together because Ray was trying to get them out of the jars with a spoon that was too large. I thought I might be getting as "crazy" as Ray, mixing this strange brew. It didn't taste too bad.

Things haven't changed much recently. Ray wanders around the house, might try to cook or make a sandwich, but usually can't. He is often bored and will come to be with someone in the house. He continues to need help dressing because he puts things on backwards and can't select the clothing he needs. He often needs guidance to the bathroom; verbal directions don't work. We had a very sad conversation the other day. I told Ray that our carpets were to be cleaned and that we should get out for the day.

RAY: Let's go to New York.
ME: How?
RAY: Subway.

ME: We can't go by subway, Honey. We have to go by plane or car.

RAY: Costs less than $5.00.

ME: Could we take the subway from here?

RAY: Yes, well, I haven't gone in a long time. Haven't been there since we lived closer than Bridgeport.

ME: Where do we live now?

RAY: Not closer than Bridgeport.

ME: What state are we in?

RAY: We live further than Milford [Connecticut].

ME: We live in North Carolina, Honey.

RAY: Oh, yeah. That's just a minor confusion. Let me try and think what state we live in. [A long pause.] We don't live in any of those states. We lived in Milford or closer to there a while ago. Didn't we?

ME: Come here, Honey. I want to hold you. [Ray came over. I held him and started to cry.]

RAY: I don't want you to feel sorry for me.

ME: I don't. [He stroked and hugged me.]

RAY: There's more here than you think.

NINE

Michael was home for the summer. Though he had to work a good deal of the time, he was there to help some. One night he came to me and told me that I needed to rely on him more. I should let him know when I wanted to go out, and he would plan to be home. He told me how helpless he felt, but said he would always be there for me. I told him that he wouldn't and shouldn't. It was Daddy I was losing, and he couldn't fill that loss. He was my child, not my husband, and although I did not want to lose him, I would have to learn to live with the loss of Daddy. I assured him that I would be okay and that he shouldn't be too concerned about my tears. I had learned that the ability to cry, to cleanse, to relieve pain, was a blessing. As long as I could get up again, and get on with life as best I could, my tears were okay and his were, too.

One day in June Ray watched the "Phil Donahue Show." Seymour Hersh was on discussing his new book, *The Price of Power*, an account of the manuevers of Nixon adviser Henry Kissinger. Ray was intrigued and said he was going to get the book. It certainly was a book Ray would have loved to have read in the past. But now he read nothing. He would turn the pages of a magazine, but his concentration and comprehension were so poor that he could not sustain more than a line or two. I didn't say anything about the book, figuring he would forget it. But he didn't.

The book was a twenty-dollar hardcover. I tried to discourage him without hurting him. I suggested he try reading something less taxing first, to see how he would do. But he insisted that he wanted the book and was really hurt when he found me to be so contrary. He felt that I didn't believe or trust in him. Even two days after the program, Ray was still talking about the book. At

Rocuth Houk

Boow wtn Gray

Ray was attempting to transcribe a phone message: "Ruth Houck—Bowman Gray [Hospital]."

788 4269

Mar Jorie Ross

A few days later, he attempted to write "Marjorie Roth." The phone number is incorrectly transcribed.

the pool that day I mentioned that I had brought a book to read. He said he didn't have anything to read. I knew that he was referring to Hersh's book.

And so on Father's Day, a few days later, we gave Ray *The Price of Power* by Seymour Hersh. It sat on the end of his night table. I remember seeing him look through the book once. But we all agreed that it was money well spent.

Even though going to the city swimming pool was one of the few things Ray and I could still do, I was always nervous. He didn't notice things like his bathing suit falling down, but if I attempted to help him hike it up, he would push me away. His limited sense of social proprieties was sufficient enough for him to know that other people don't adjust your pants, at least not in public. Even though nobody probably paid any attention,

I was very conscious of what the two of us must have looked like to anyone watching.

When Ray forgot how to get wet in the water, I would take both his hands and try to get him to bounce, bending his knees. Once he began in this way, the memory would often return, and he would be able to enjoy the water, remembering how to float and even do a crawl.

He wanted to dive in the water. Just like the mother of a young child, I would have to tell him to use the steps. I was always afraid he might make a scene, and I was afraid to take my eyes off of him in the pool. Gradually, I began to realize that Ray didn't enjoy the water as he used to. He complained about noise and kids splashing. He never had liked sitting in the hot sun and would spend most of the time in the water. Now he didn't seem to even know that he was hot and uncomfortable when he was out of the water. Even when he was in the water, he usually just stood up to his waist so that he barely cooled off. One afternoon he told me, "I'm just not as spontaneous in the water as I used to be." We stopped going to the pool. Sometimes I would go alone, but we never went together again.

Betty and Barbara, two old friends I had worked with in Connecticut, came to visit for a few days, and their visit proved to be an important turning point. I was very apprehensive about their coming. Other people had seen Ray, but we could usually prepare for their visits. Ray was able to handle being with people for short periods of time without showing the severity of his problems. But with people staying at our house for three days, we could not escape the inevitable. I did not want Ray to feel demeaned. I did not want my friends to be uncomfortable, and I did not want to feel torn between my desire to be with them and feelings of abandoning Ray.

Part of me wanted to protect and cover for Ray, while another part of me wanted them to know about his condition. I wanted them to see what life was really like for us now, partly, I guess, for them to provide some support and understanding, but also to help give me some needed perspective. And they were able to do that.

If Betty and Barbara had come at a time when Ray was well, the three of us would have spent a good deal of time alone—shopping, going out to lunch, sightseeing. But it was different now. I could not leave Ray.

The four of us went to lunch one afternoon. I had to guide Ray from the car to the restaurant, lead him to a seat, and help him sit down. He was not able to read or understand the menu, and so I ordered for him. He had some difficulty eating his meal and barely said anything during the entire afternoon. Betty, Barbara, and I laughed about old times. They brought me up to date about the people we had known and what was happening in their lives. We tried each others' lunch orders and indulged in sinful desserts, vowing not to eat anything for dinner.

But it wasn't relaxed. I was always on my guard, never knowing what to expect. They must have felt my anxiety plus their own apprehension. I wished Ray were not with us and yet felt terrible that I could think that. But it was true. He would not have come if he were well. It was a time for old friends to be together.

After lunch I took Barbara and Betty to some of the shops in Reynolda Village, a nearby shopping area. We were in a bookstore when Ray told me, quite urgently, that he had to go to the bathroom "right now." I knew I had better act fast. I quickly went to a woman at the counter and asked if there was a restroom in the store. She directed us to one. We had no problem because I was able to go with Ray. But I realized that to take Ray out in public meant I had to consider his inability to anticipate when he would need to go to the bathroom, as well as plan so that he did not have to go in alone.

I decided that I needed to spend some time alone with Betty and Barbara. We planned dinner the next evening with another friend of mine. It was the first time that I would be leaving Ray for something other than an obligatory meeting. Michael was to be home at 7 P.M. He and Ray would have dinner together.

When Ray saw the three of us starting to get ready at about

6 : 30, he went to his closet. He asked me what he should wear. My heart was heavy as I told him, in as casual a voice as I could muster, that just the three of us were going. I said it was "a night out with the girls," but I could tell he wanted to go and didn't understand why he couldn't.

By seven we were ready to leave. Part of me wanted to just forget it. I was filled with guilt at "abandoning" Ray, but I knew I just couldn't bring him. When Michael came home, I reasoned, Ray would be fine. My friends and I waited outside a few minutes for Michael. Ray came out and waited, too, somewhat confused about what was happening. I just wanted to get out of there. I couldn't stand watching Ray be so left-out. I wanted Michael to come home and was getting more and more upset when he didn't. I knew he hadn't forgotten and would be there any minute. But it seemed like an eternity. Ray looked so pathetic. I could barely stand it. We got into the car, hoping Michael would pull up, hoping Ray would go inside. But Michael didn't come and Ray didn't go in.

Michael arrived at 7 : 15. He had been trying to find the Nova Scotia salmon that Ray liked so much and had gone to a number of stores without luck. By that time, I was so emotionally drained from the experience that I burst into tears. I didn't want to spoil the others' evening, and since I had already committed myself, I wanted to have a good time as well. But it took a while for the tears to stop and for me to compose myself, trying very hard to get into the spirit of what I hoped would turn out to have a better ending than its beginning. It turned out to be a delightful evening. We spent the evening at a downtown outdoor restaurant. We ate, drank, talked, and for a few hours I felt some release.

The evening helped me gain a somewhat different perspective. I knew that Ray was in good hands with Michael and would not dwell on my being gone. I needed to try to overcome my guilt. If Ray had been his old self, he would have told me to go, enjoy myself, make the best of it. I tried to let the words penetrate. I tried to allow my many past conversations with Ray to help guide and direct my course.

I was finally ready to look for someone to help Ray. I decided to start by putting an ad in the local paper. My plan was to try to get someone to live with us in exchange for free housing. In return that person would be available to Ray during the hours I was at work. I thought perhaps an older person—a writer or craftsperson, perhaps—would be interested. If I couldn't get live-in help, then perhaps I could find someone who would like a place to work and could also be available during the day for Ray. My ad must have sounded strange, but I needed to see what kind of response I might get.

I received responses from only three people, none of whom would have provided Ray with what he needed. One was a woman who wrote a very syrupy letter about how her heart went out to us, how she would love to help care for a person whose life she could help brighten. I knew that wouldn't work. I needed someone who could help Ray retain as much self-respect as possible; someone who wouldn't radiate pity—who would care, and yet remain a bit detached. The other two people who responded had jobs with irregular hours and could not be consistently available when I had to be away from home. I was gradually facing the fact that someone needed to be with Ray all the time.

During Betty and Barbara's visit, Marjorie called to tell me about the arrangements that had been made at Duke. Ray was scheduled to be admitted July 10. He would be in the hospital one week. I was to bring all of the records that I had obtained, including the CAT scan that was done almost two years before.

July 3

Ray told the kids today that he didn't have anything to his name anymore. When I asked him what he meant he said that he had seen an insurance policy and his name wasn't on it. No such thing occurred.

His sense of time is so poor that he cannot delay having his needs met. We plan to go to Seabrook Island in South Carolina at the beginning of August. Ray keeps asking when we're going and thinks I am postponing it. He gets very frustrated when I tell him it's not time yet. The same kind of problem arose the other day. He saw a picture of Shelly Long, the actress on the TV program "Cheers." He immediately wanted to watch the program. He spent a lot of time trying to tune the program in at a time and day when it wasn't on. He just didn't understand.

Although Ray continues to have great difficult expressing himself, so much specific information remains intact. I was reading something and came across the word "epistemology." I asked him if he knew what it meant. He said, "It means how you know the things you know. It's used specifically in referring to knowledge and knowledge systems." A few minutes later, however, he told me his sandwich was stuck to the table and he couldn't move it.

Early in the summer I would plan to do errands in the morning while David was home. When Michael would go to work, David would have to look after Ray by himself. But I realized I was finding more and more reasons to stay away for longer periods, leaving David with the responsibility of caring for his father. I knew he wouldn't leave Ray until I came home, and I knew once I was home, I wouldn't be able to get away.

At dinner one evening the issue came to a head. David and Michael argued quite openly about what they each expected of the other. David did not blame me. I think he was torn between his wanting to be free of this burdensome responsibility and his love for Ray and understanding of my own imprisonment. So he attacked Michael, accusing him of not being more available. David felt that our family should come first, even above Michael's summer job. Michael protested, arguing that he needed to work. The turmoil my two boys were feeling poignantly reinforced my determination to get help. I knew I was putting it off. I detested the idea of some stranger coming into our home, taking care of my husband. How would Ray feel about that? How would we handle it? I had resented and fought it for much too long. I could no longer rationalize that we were managing.

July 4

Ray told me the other day that I deny him everything. When I asked him for an example, he told me that I wouldn't let him drive. He knew he could still drive. Later in the day he told me that he thought that a good thing for him to do would be to go to law school. I didn't know how to respond to him.

Later that evening, we talked with Lily and Rich. He told them his plan. It was so sad listening to him tell Rich that he thought that entering law school would help change his life.

Ray continued to have occasional interest in sex, but I just didn't think I could handle it. I found that if I put if off awhile, he forgot. I felt guilty denying him that, but always found it so frustrating and unfulfilling that I tried to avoid it, even though I missed it desperately.

One evening early in July I couldn't stand it any longer. What was already a purely physical, poorly executed act became sheer emptiness that night. Ray was completely unable to participate as a sex partner. I knew I could never make love to Ray again. I couldn't bear the frustration and anguish it evoked. A part of me died that night. Another piece of our life together was gone. What was left?

The next day Ray got up and wandered around the house. He was unable to talk. His speech was garbled and, except for isolated words, unintelligible. He knew that he could not speak, and when I asked him if that upset him he said, "Mildly." It lasted about twenty minutes.

I abandoned my other ideas on how to provide home care for Ray. I decided that the most practical thing to do would be to rent out the downstairs and use that income to help pay for someone to come in to stay with Ray during the day. I began to let people know I was looking for someone, and although I did not have many leads, I did get a few.

Adam was the first man I hired. He was recommended to me by a friend who had known him for a number of years. He started in July on a part-time basis so that he could get to know Ray, and so that Ray would get used to having someone else in the house. I would be home most of the time, but Adam would come in for a few hours a day.

Adam was a tall, large man of close to forty. He lived with his mother and worked part-time in a beauty supply house as a stock clerk, but was available most of the day. He loved sports and was an avid Atlanta Braves fan. He drove, and had taken some group trips abroad that he talked about with obvious pleasure and fond memories. However, he had never taken care of or been responsible for another person.

Adam was insecure about this new challenge, but very much wanted to meet it. He bent over backwards to do everything possible for Ray. But, in spite of Ray's limited judgment and insight, he was aware of and irritated by Adam's deferential and servile manner. Although Ray recognized Adam's sincere attempts to be helpful, he told me, "He's obsequious. He panders." Somehow Ray sensed that he was not safe and once said of Adam, "I can't depend on him." When asked, though, if he thought it better not to have Adam around, he answered, "No, I think I need someone."

I spent some time with Adam, teaching him how to prepare some of the lunches Ray liked—egg salad, grilled cheese, and steak sandwiches. Adam worked hard to learn to do things that would please Ray. I knew that he was a kind and caring man, whom I hoped Ray would grow to trust in the same way he did his family.

The confusion never ceased. One day Ray told a friend on the phone that Adam was a student at Wake Forest University we'd hired by putting an ad in the help-wanted section. Ray had combined unrelated incidents to create this story. I had called Wake Forest, which was just two miles from our home, and had listed our downstairs apartment with student housing. Did he remember that I had placed an ad in the paper a few weeks earlier or was it just a piece of information he had added to connect the two unrelated incidents? In any case, the explanation as to how Adam entered the picture was completely inaccurate.

July 6

This afternoon David drove to the store. He still has his driver's permit so Ray and I went along. While he was in the store, Ray said, "I feel like my life is over. I can't make any decisions. But, it doesn't have to be over . . ." He was trying to open the car door, and then asked, "Why can't I open this door?" When he saw David coming out of the store, he said, "Oh look, there's little David. What's he doing there?"

July 7

I came home from the parcourse this morning to find Ray in the kitchen. Both boys were asleep. He had urinated on the steps and on the kitchen floor, but didn't know that he had. He kept talking about wanting juice. He picked up an empty juice can and told me that it was full. When I said, "I guess you had a tough morning," he said, "No, what makes you think that?"

A while later he called me into the room where he was and, pointing at the wall, said, "Where is that juice?" I said, "That isn't juice. Juice is in the kitchen."

"Did you supply it? . . . I had a great idea last night. There's a way to get rich off car places. Buy a car for money and invest it for cash."

"How do you make money?"

"Buy a car for money and invest it . . . There's a mystery around here. Everything's wet [referring to the wet carpet I had just cleaned] . . . When are we going?"

"Where, Honey?"

[Angry] "Aren't we going anywhere?"

"No, we weren't planning to. I tutor in a half hour. Where did you want to go?"

"Okay. If you want to play games, I will too."

Another day Ray returned to the idea of making money by acquiring a car. The kids and I couldn't help but be hysterical even though Ray was quite serious. Ray said, "I have an idea to buy a new car for our use and sell it. We should buy it immediately and it will be an investment. We'd have to pay about $3000, close to $3000. So it would wind up costing us about $3200. The price would depend on the temperature."

July 8

Ray was quiet today. He seemed depressed, but when I asked, he said he didn't know why. This evening I allowed myself to feel how much I miss him. I was walking home from the Douglases' across the street. It was a beautiful evening, cool and peaceful, and I remembered similar evenings when I could take Ray's hand and feel so good being with him; happy, content, lucky that we were together. But that's no more, never will be, and I miss him terribly; miss his touch, that look of understanding between two people who know each other so well, the knowledge that he'll be there, my friend, my lover. He's gone. Instead, I helplessly watch him deteriorate, move further and further away from me. I'm afraid that if it goes on, my memories will be replaced by the images before me now.

TEN

On July 10, Ray was admitted to the giant North Hospital of the world-famous Duke University Medical Center in Durham, N.C. He would remain there for two weeks—a period in which he, and I, would variously be confused, frightened, infuriated, and relieved. The physicians at Duke were able to find out at last what was happening to Ray—but not before both of us had experienced the bureaucratic disorientation of a huge, impersonal hospital.

When Ray arrived, a resident took an extensive medical history. Although Ray appeared to understand where he was, and seemed to experience no more confusion than usual, he was unable to give much accurate information. I explained Ray's impaired state to the nurse, tried to give her some idea of the problems I thought he might encounter in the hospital, and answered the questions she had asked him.

I left the hospital about 7 P.M. I was somewhat concerned about what the nurses knew about Ray. I knew he would be quiet and would not ask for anything; but he did not know how to use the call button if he needed help. He might not know how to find the bathroom. Although I hated to deny him one of his few pleasures, I decided to put his lighter away when I wasn't there—at least that wouldn't be a problem.

When I arrived the next morning, I found Ray very alert and responsive. Speaking of the hospital, he said, "What I would suggest is that we establish a working relationship." I asked what he meant and he answered, "You know. Bypass all the red tape. I realize that every new situation has its traps—all these new people, pharmacy . . ." Then he lost the thought.

The doctors assigned to Ray's case were Dr. Byron Holmes, a

neurologist who worked closely with Dr. Hindle, and Dr. Storm, a neurology resident. That morning I met Dr. Storm, who would be on the floor during the day. I had brought all the records that I was responsible for; but now I was told that Dr. Storm and Dr. Holmes had not received any of the hospital records that were sent from Winston-Salem. I was very upset. Marjorie had sent those records well in advance of Ray's hospitalization. I expected the doctors to have already reviewed Ray's case and have some plans about how to proceed. I called Dr. Holmes's office and found that Dr. Holmes had received the records three days earlier, but had not yet reviewed them.

Shortly after I talked with his secretary, Dr. Holmes came to Ray's room. He was a medium-sized man, dark, soft-spoken. He asked me to step out into the hall. According to the secretary with whom I had just spoken, Dr. Holmes had not reviewed Ray's medical history. But now he told me Ray probably had Alzheimer's disease. I was furious! On what evidence did he say that—not knowing me, or what I might or might not know about Alzheimer's disease? He went on to say that he had not read the records yet and that he could not really answer any questions. He asked me what I thought the onset of early symptoms had been and what Ray's IQ had originally been. I answered the questions as best I could, but my confidence in Dr. Holmes, at least from this initial meeting, was near zero.

From the Alzheimer's support group in Winston-Salem I had learned of the Duke Center for Aging, which was also the headquarters for the North Carolina Alzheimer's Disease and Related Disorders Association (ADRDA) chapter, providing organization, information, and workshops to family support group affiliates in North Carolina. My friend Jan had come to Durham with me. We went to the center and met a specialist named Laura Miller.

Laura told us about research programs that were going on at Duke, and then explained Medicare coverage if Ray should need it. (After being on Social Security disability for two years, an individual is eligible for Medicare, even if he has not yet reached his sixty-fifth birthday.) She gave us some information about nursing facilities and discussed some research concerning language changes associated with dementia.

After we met with Laura, Jan and I viewed a videotape that had been shown on educational television. It was titled *Someone I Once Knew* and presented a series of Alzheimer's victims who were in various stages of the disease. Riveting our attention, as if we were actually living with a victim, the film tore at our hearts. There was one interview with a victim's wife who reminded me very much of myself. She quoted two lines from Robert Browning's poem "Rabbi Ben Ezra": "Grow old with me!/ The best is yet to be!" She knew that would never be for her. I knew it would never be for me.

We were away from Ray for about two hours. When we returned, the door was open, but the curtain was drawn around his bed. I could see Ray's shadow behind the curtain, and I knew something was wrong. Ray was standing next to the bed wearing a hospital gown. He saw me and grew furious. "How could you leave me?" he demanded. "You were gone two and a half hours. I needed you, and you weren't here." Under the angry tone, I could hear the agony and desperation in his voice.

While we were gone, Ray had gone into the bathroom and defecated on the floor. He had left the bathroom, tracking feces into the room, before someone came to his rescue. He was mortified. I held him in my arms for a while and it seemed to help, but he remained angry at me and embarrassed by the incident. I helped him dress in street clothes, which I felt would help reestablish some of his feeling of dignity, and then we took a walk around the hospital floor. Ray referred to the incident a number of times after that—even a month or two later. It still makes me ache for him every time I think of it.

After this humiliating experience, I tried to meet each of the nurses who came into contact with Ray. I wanted to explain that he needed to be checked frequently, since he would not know how to seek help should he need it. There were many nurses involved due to shift changes, and I was never really sure how seriously they took me.

July 12

I got to the hospital about 9:30 this morning. An LPN was reading the choices for tomorrow's meals to Ray. I'm sure she must have been having a difficult time, since Ray had trouble holding the choices in his head long enough to select his preference. He is at a point that he really can't make a decision between two foods, even if he could remember them.

Ray was sitting on a chair in a hospital gown. He had been wearing pajamas when I left, but the nurse said that he had wet the bed. Ray did not appear upset, but when she left he began to stare vacantly into space. When I asked him what was wrong he said that he didn't like having these "difficulties" and that he was really upset with me. He felt abandoned, that he was left to fend for himself. I explained that I just couldn't be there all the time and that I knew it was hard for him. I asked if he wanted to get dressed. He said he did. When I asked him to shave and brush his teeth, handing him the toothbrush first, he refused by saying I was "too fussy." I didn't push it, but five minutes later asked him again. This time he willingly obliged. But he remained depressed throughout the morning.

I believed that Ray's feelings of being abandoned were really his acknowledgment of his dependency and semi-awareness of what was happening to him. Although I felt some guilt, I knew that I couldn't do much better and stay in reasonable mental shape. I didn't feel I should talk to him about it much because that would only make it worse. Talking things through the way we had in the past was no longer an aspect of our relationship. I counted on the disease to destroy his awareness. It was the only compensation for the destruction of his mind.

I did tell Ray that I thought it was good that we had come to Duke and that maybe they could help us. I tried to act positive without lying or giving false promises. But watching him just stare into space I knew how depressed he must have been and wondered what I could say. What should I have told him?

Ray was at Duke two full days before a CAT scan was performed. Dr. Storm said that his office had not received the records of other CAT scans. When I asked what else was planned, he didn't seem to know. I was becoming very anxious. So far, all Ray had had were problems and nothing seemed to be happening.

On the second day, I approached Dr. Storm in the hall and asked him if he had contacted Dr. Holmes yet to see about the CAT scan. He said he hadn't. I tried to keep calm, but I was about to explode, not so much from anger as from frustration. We had wasted two days in the hospital, I told him; a CAT scan could have been done before Ray ever checked in. Dr. Storm reacted to my urgency with a condescending air; but he said that he would check as soon as he was finished with his patient.

In the two days that Ray had spent in the hospital, he had experienced humiliation, abandonment, and some level of awareness of his plight. I had assumed that the doctors on the case would have reviewed all the records by the time he entered the hospital, and would have had some plan for proceeding. But, in fact, that was not the situation. Jan had gone back to Winston for a day, and I had no one even to let off steam to.

I came back to Ray's room, closed the door and cried. I could be strong, do what had to be done. But inside I desperately needed to be cared for and relieved of this consuming emotional exhaustion. Crying was often my only release. Ray was asleep, but heard me crying and awoke. "What's the matter, Honey?" he asked in a way that was like a voice from the past. I walked over to the bed and put my head on his chest. "Hold me?" I asked. He put his arms around me, confused as usual by my state of mind. Then he fell back to sleep.

A few minutes later Dr. Storm came back into the room. It was obvious that I had been crying; he appeared more responsive and sensitive. He said that he was missing the psychological testing. I found copies of the testing results he needed and told him of the arrangements for getting copies of the previous CAT scans.

Late that afternoon Dr. Storm passed by Ray's room, saw me, and came in. We talked a bit about a possible lumbar puncture to check for infection. This procedure entails taking a specimen of cerebrospinal fluid from the lumbar region at the base of the spine. As he was leaving, Dr. Storm said matter-of-factly that Ray had wandered into another unit the night before. Someone had found him and brought him back. "Okay?" he asked as he got ready to go.

Surprising myself, I responded, "No, it's not okay." He retraced his steps, entering the doorway again. I proceeded to tell him about the need to have the nursing staff know more about Ray; he wandered, couldn't find the bathroom, didn't know how to call for help. I recounted the unpleasant experiences he had had and now the fact that he had wandered into another part of the hospital. His problems were different from those of most patients on the floor. Dr. Storm said he would relay my concerns to the nurses. I didn't think of it then, but should have said, "They should be *your* concerns." I've always been great with the comebacks after the fact.

Ray finally went for a CAT scan the evening of his second day in the hospital. On the third day I arrived at 7:30 A.M. to make sure I would see Dr. Holmes to get the results. Ray welcomed me with a smile and said, "About time you got here." Then he retreated into silent depression. Later in the morning I told Ray to trust that I would take care of him. I would be his advocate even when I was not there. He looked at me impatiently and said, "I don't care about that."

"What do you care about, Honey?"

"I care about peeing. I care about peeing."

Dr. Holmes arrived and said that the scan didn't show any atrophy, which is often found in the CAT scans of Alzheimer's victims, but it did show considerable loss of the brain's white matter (the tissue that contains fibers connecting brain cells) and small areas representing infarctions—small areas of tissue that had died because of blocked blood supply. He believed that Ray never had normal pressure hydrocephalus; instead, the doctors now suspected that Ray had multi-infarct dementia.

163

Ray was having numerous small infarcts, or strokes, that were destroying brain cells. I had read about multi-infarct dementia and knew it to be second to Alzheimer's disease as the cause of dementia. Like Alzheimer's disease, it was incurable and progressive.

Dr. Holmes also said that he had become concerned because Ray's heart murmur was quite pronounced. Although the heart murmur had been considered serious, it had not prevented him from participating in any activities as a child, but had earned him a 4-F draft classification. Dr. Holmes said that an echocardiogram (which reads the heart's action using ultrasound) would be scheduled and that a cardiologist would see Ray.

Dr. Holmes was especially interested in the numerous times Ray had experienced numbness and dizziness. He also asked if there seemed to be periods of plateauing, in which Ray would be better or the same for a period of time, then deteriorate quickly and level off again for a while. I said that did not seem to be the pattern. Ray seemed to be showing steady, relatively rapid deterioration. Even though there were periods in which he seemed improved, they never lasted.

Dr. Holmes concluded by telling me that Ray should stop smoking right away. Smoking was only making things worse for him.

Ray willingly threw his cigarettes away that morning when I told him what the doctor had said. But in my mind, I was asking him to do it for safety reasons, not because I thought it would have any significant, or even temporary, effect on his condition. I also knew that even though he seemed alert enough to know what he was doing, he wouldn't remember that he had agreed to stop smoking.

After Ray had been in the hospital for four days, Dr. Holmes told me he believed that Ray had some arteriosclerosis. The CAT scan showed that his brain density was low at the juncture of the white matter with the gray matter, which contains most of the neurons, or brain cells. He said the changes were asymmetrical—affecting one side more than the other—which is typically seen in multi-infarct dementia rather than in Alzheimer's. Although Dr. Holmes had not ruled out Alzheimer's disease, there was no evidence of the brain's atrophying, or shrinking, as is usually seen in Alzheimer's victims.

A few days later, Dr. Holmes returned with an entourage of neurology residents. He asked Ray a lot of questions.

"Where do you live?"

"Brighton Beach." (Ray had lived in Brighton Beach fifteen years earlier.)

"What do you do for a living?"

"I'm an architect. I make my living as an architect. My profession is . . ." (There was a long pause; then he lost his train of thought.)

"Where is Brighton Beach?"

"Northern part of state." (Brighton Beach is at the southern tip of Brooklyn.)

"What county?"

"Kings."

"Are you married?"

"Yes."

"What is your wife's name?"

"Myrna."

"Do you have any children?"

"Yes."

"How many?" (Ray thought a long while.) "Three. David . . ." (He couldn't remember Michael's name).

"What is your problem?"

"I have memory problems."

"How does that affect you?"

Ray was unable to answer the question.

Then Dr. Holmes did a series of neurological tests, checking grasp reflexes. He had Ray walk, turn, and walk with one foot directly in front of the other. His gait wasn't too bad, but he had a lot of trouble walking with one foot in front of the other.

As Jan and I were leaving Ray's room to get a soda from the hospital cafeteria, she spotted a small object on the floor underneath the edge of the bed. It was a tiny starfish. I thought it might have been washed ashore from the Brighton Beach where Ray was living in his mind.

Dr. Kutcher, a cardiologist, came to see Ray. From his examination it appeared that Ray had a more severe heart problem than was initially suspected. The infarcts in the brain might even be stemming from the heart problem. Dr. Kutcher mentioned a possible need for another heart catheterization. This time a catheterization would entail the use of dye, which would put Ray's kidneys at risk. If the catheterization found serious heart disease, Ray would need extensive surgery, during which he'd be placed on a heart-lung machine. This, too, would put his kidneys in great danger. Even if both procedures were successful, the best we could hope for would be to arrest the disease. There would not be any improvement. What was the quality of Ray's life now? What would he have chosen?

If we did nothing, though, Ray would probably continue to have multiple infarcts—perhaps a larger stroke, Dr. Kutcher said. If the problem was in his heart, he might go into cardiac arrest.

I was overwhelmed by these life-or-death decisions. I left the hospital about 8:30 that evening. I called the boys, told them the situation and the decisions we might face. Then I called Marjorie. I didn't get her until about 10 P.M., and by that time, I was over some of the initial impact and beginning to think more clearly. But Marjorie could provide me with some medical insight, as well as help me as a friend. I explained the findings and possible conclusions. Marjorie said frankly that she would not go ahead with anything. There was too much risk and too little to gain.

When I got off the phone, I felt better. Marjorie had confirmed my thinking. If the doctors recommended a heart catheterization, I would have to weigh the risks against any possible gain. Based on what I knew now, I would not consent.

The next morning I met Dr. Holmes during rounds. He had spoken with Dr. Kutcher and decided to do a Muga scan as an initial procedure. He told me it was a safe procedure in which a radioisotope is injected, allowing doctors to assess the functioning of the heart. In addition, for twenty-four hours, Ray would wear a monitor that would take a cardiogram. Ray would be released the next day, but some additional information needed to be gathered first. Dr. Holmes contradicted Dr. Kutcher: it was unlikely that Ray would have a major stroke. Depending on the activity and rhythm of the heart, medication might be recommended, and perhaps a pacemaker. But no further mention was made of a heart catheterization. That solved one problem.

I had talked with Dr. Holmes earlier about a pre-mortem consent form. Whatever Ray had could better, and perhaps only, be diagnosed upon autopsy. It was important to me and our children (and I knew would have been to Ray) to have some concrete answers eventually. Ray was an organ donor, and had no concerns about how his body should be disposed of upon death. I knew that signing permission for an autopsy was not a binding commitment. I could change my mind, but I was pretty sure I wouldn't. Still, it was better to do it now, rather than wait for perhaps a more difficult time.

Ray went down for the Muga scan in mid-morning. I stayed on the floor, chatting with the patient in the next room and tried not to worry. About an hour after they had taken Ray down, Dr. Storm called the nurses' station and asked to speak with me. He told me that while they were doing the scan, an abnormality in Ray's heart rate had occurred. Ray's sinoatrial node, which is the heart's natural pacemaker, was not firing. He was asymptomatic, showing no signs that his pulse had dropped to thirty-three. He had experienced no pain and did not realize that anything was wrong.

Dr. Storm called to tell me that they were transferring Ray to the cardiac care floor to monitor his heart. Perhaps a pacemaker would be needed.

I remembered when a first-degree block had been found in Ray's heart about two years before. Then in February, Ray had undergone a heart catheterization before surgery, because doctors had found a second-degree block. Now, it was a third-degree block. We were not going home tomorrow.

They brought Ray to the Cardiac Care Unit (CCU) and hooked him up to a monitor. The nurse, Connie, helped make Ray comfortable. Unlike the nurses on the neurology floor, she seemed instinctively to be in tune to Ray's needs and limitations. Because he was in an intensive care unit, he would be monitored much more carefully. Connie would be his nurse on the three-to-eleven shift, and I knew he would be well cared-for.

Shortly after Ray arrived, Dr. Holmes called me into the hall. He found two stools in back of an empty nurses' station and invited me to sit down. He reviewed the findings thus far, and said that his best-educated guess was that Ray had multi-infarct dementia. He had a heart problem, perhaps related, perhaps not, to the dementia.

Then quite unexpectedly he told me that I needed to leave Ray more. He encouraged me to get sitters and go out with friends. His tone was warm and fatherly. It was the first time that I had sensed any real emotion from him, and I welcomed it. "Otherwise, you will lose your friends," he went on. "Ray doesn't need you as much as you think." He continued by telling me that they planned to put in a temporary pacemaker that day and after the weekend would implant a permanent pacemaker.

He knew my parents were coming to Winston-Salem that afternoon since we had planned to go home by then. He encouraged me to leave that afternoon, go home for the weekend, and return to Duke on Monday.

I did as he suggested. I knew that Connie, Ray's three-to-eleven shift nurse, would be on duty through the weekend. And, because he was in a cardiac care unit, Ray would be carefully watched. He was hooked up to a monitor and couldn't get out of bed. If I didn't go home, I probably wouldn't get to see my parents, who had come from Florida. I needed a break. I explained my plans to Ray and to Connie, instructing her to call if Ray needed me.

I drove the hour and a half from Durham to Winston-Salem feeling surprisingly relaxed. I was anxious to see my parents who had been so supportive throughout these long and difficult months. The Durham community offered a host program to people who came to visit a hospitalized friend or relative, and I had arranged for my parents to stay with one of the host families. We would all return on Sunday afternoon.

That weekend I drove a little with David, who needed me to be in the car so that he could practice prior to getting his license. I did some much-needed laundry, got a haircut, and spent some time with my parents. Marjorie and Stuart came over one evening.

My parents and I returned on Sunday afternoon. As we entered the hospital, we bumped into Connie who was just getting off duty. She said that Ray had slept well and was better oriented, but was feeling abandoned. In fact, she said she had called me at my home, but we had left already. The doctors had decided not to put in a temporary pacemaker.

When we entered Ray's room, he was sitting in a chair and recognized my parents immediately. But as time passed, he became quieter and more distant.

New people were becoming involved in Ray's case now. First was Dr. Kingsley, who was a cardiology resident. He explained that no final decision had been made on the pacemaker, and went on to say that he did not feel that the heart problem was related to the dementia. The problem with Ray's heart was probably related to the rheumatic fever that he had had as a child. He said that the sinoatrial node was not strong enough to get the blood out of the aorta and into the heart, thereby limiting the blood supply.

That afternoon the doctors did a blood-gas test to check the oxygen in the blood. It must have been very painful because Ray remembered and talked about it for days.

Dr. Kingsley was doing rounds in the CCU when I saw him the next morning. I waited outside Ray's door to see what they would say. So many people were now involved in the case that I didn't know who Ray's primary care physician was anymore. Dr. Holmes was temporarily out of the picture because Ray was under cardiac care. So I tried to get information from whoever seemed to be in charge.

Dr. Kingsley said that Dr. Kutcher planned to have a permanent pacemaker implanted the next day. I asked what would happen if Ray didn't have a pacemaker. Dr. Kingsley suggested that I talk to Dr. Kutcher about that. He said that they weren't sure if a pacemaker would improve Ray's condition, but a weak heartbeat could impede blood flow.

I called Dr. Kutcher's office to discuss the pacemaker with him. I asked what would happen if we elected not to have it implanted. I didn't want to put Ray through anything needlessly, and, at this point, I had doubts about procedures that would prolong his life without improving his mental status. Dr. Kutcher said that without a pacemaker Ray might develop symptoms of heart disease: dizziness, blackouts, and more problems in the brain. The block could become severe enough to cause a heart attack. He did not believe, however, that the heart problem was causing the dementia, and he felt it was very questionable whether the pacemaker would help his mental status. It was impossible to know how much of the problem in the brain was permanent and how much was temporary.

Although the only promise the doctors could make was that Ray's heart would beat at a normal rhythm, I decided to go ahead. Implantation of a pacemaker is a relatively simple procedure, and I felt I could not deny Ray the benefits of it.

My parents and I went down to the cafeteria for lunch. I had been trying to listen carefully, understand what was happening, and prepare for what decisions might have to be made. But at lunch I began to let down and talk about how I was feeling. I had learned to function without feeling, and when I let down my defenses, fear and desperation closed in on me. I was tired of bearing up to pain and anxiety. The tears began to run down my cheeks. My father, usually so strong and stoic, started to cry, and then my mother. There we were, in the middle of the hospital cafeteria during a crowded lunch hour, crying. I put my arms around my father and told him not to worry, that I'd survive this. I'd be okay. Ray would want me to be happy again, and I would be.

I can imagine how hard it must have been for my parents to watch me in such pain. I was beginning to know that feeling myself. As my boys were getting older, I was no longer able to intercede in their lives the way I could when they were younger. Taking them in my arms and drying their tears wasn't enough any longer. They were learning to deal with their own hurts, their own mistakes, their own problems. It was an inevitable part of becoming a mature adult. But as a parent, I found it difficult to let go, to watch them struggle, grope, make mistakes. I knew how my parents were feeling that afternoon and knew, probably for the first time in my life, how shared pain can strengthen the bonds between family members.

That afternoon my parents and I went to Duke Gardens, wandered around a shopping mall for a while, and then went to Chapel Hill for dinner. When we got back to the hospital Ray was asleep, but got up to eat. He said he was in a good mood and when I asked why, he said, "Because the surgery is over." I asked him, "What surgery?" and he answered, "The pacemaker."

"It's not over yet, Honey."

"It is for me."

The pacemaker procedure was done in what was called the "electrophysiology room." It took about two and a half hours. Ray was given Novocain and a Valium IV, but was awake throughout. The pacemaker, which was about the size of a pack of cigarettes, was placed just under the skin over the heart. It was a dual-chambered-type pacemaker and was set to make sure Ray's heart beat at sixty beats per minute. If his natural heartbeat dropped below sixty, then the pacemaker would take over. He had some mild pain after the Novocain wore off, but there were no problems or other discomforts.

Before my parents and I left the hospital that evening, Ray asked me, "When are you having your procedure done?" And then in the next breath, he said he was really ready to get well and believed that if he started to eat and drink well, he would recover.

The next few days in the hospital were unremarkable. Ray was anxious to go home. He sometimes seemed to understand what had happened, but remained quiet. One night he asked what was for dinner. I told him that it was chicken breast Hawaiian. He said, "That sounds risky." "Why does that sound risky, Honey?" I asked. Ray answered, "It could be bad or it could be terrible."

Another time he commented from out of the blue, "It's too bad I can't remember where my favorite supermarkets are. I could go there and get the favorite things I like."

Ray was sitting in a chair one afternoon when he said, "Could you push me over to . . . Do you know where I want to go?"

"No."

"Maybe it'll occur to me."

Dr. Hindle came to see us a couple of times. Once he saw me alone. We met for what seemed like a long time, and he asked me a lot of questions, trying to find out about the past course of Ray's illness. He was also interested in what Ray was still able to do. Could he sweep a floor? Set a table? Make a cup of coffee? Dress himself? The answer to each question was "no."

Dr. Hindle also did some brief tests of Ray's remote and recent memory. Ray did not know how old he was, nor did he know the day of the week, the month, or the year. He did recognize the name of the hospital, but initially did not know what schools he had attended. Later he remembered attending Brooklyn College and Pratt Institute. He thought World War II had begun in 1944 and had ended in 1954. But Dr. Hindle was able to see the pockets of information that were still preserved. Ray volunteered the correct name of the naval commander of Pearl Harbor during World War II. He remembered that Roosevelt was president during that time. He knew that Reagan was our present president, but did not remember the previous one.

Dr. Hindle gave Ray a name and address to remember, but

when he asked him to repeat it after a two-minute waiting period, Ray could not recall either. Ray couldn't count backward from twenty beyond ten and was unable to subtract three from 100. Even in simple addition of threes, he made gross errors.

Ray did not seem disturbed by the memory loss that he appeared to recognize. But as Dr. Hindle was leaving, Ray asked, "Is there any hope for me?" The doctor answered, "Yes, sure."

The evening before Ray was released, I spoke with Dr. Hindle again. Although he was not Ray's primary physician, I respected his national reputation and could sense a special caring quality about him. He said that he believed Ray would continue to deteriorate at the same rate, but that he didn't know for how long or how bad it would get.

I got to the hospital early the next morning. Dr. Holmes was making rounds and asked me to come into a conference room. Dr. Holmes and I sat down. The residents who accompanied him stood clustered near the closed door.

Their sober faces and my weakened emotional state made the meeting difficult. At long last, after more than a year of wandering in the dark, I heard a definite diagnosis: Ray had multi-infarct dementia—a series of small strokes were destroying his once-healthy brain, a small chunk at a time. Dr. Holmes said that Ray had a form of multi-infarct dementia called Binswanger's disease; in medical terms, subcortical arteriosclerotic encephalopathy. It is an uncommon cerebrovascular disease in which high blood pressure is usually a major cause and dementia a result. A CAT scan will reveal small strokes, a thickening of small arteries, and a diffuse pallor of the white matter. The rate of progression is unknown and there is no treatment.

I asked why we couldn't have found all this out sooner, why we had to suffer through the earlier diagnosis and the surgery to drain the fluid. He answered that, in the earlier stages of the disease, the CAT scans look very similar to normal pressure hydrocephalus. In other words, the disease doesn't reveal its distinguishing characteristics until late in the progression.

I filled out the consent form giving permission to have Ray's brain, heart, and kidneys autopsied after death. Dr. Holmes explained the procedure that I should follow in notifying the hospital. Perhaps it was premature for me to have proceeded with such arrangements, but I knew that despite all efforts, Ray's brain was deteriorating and that his case was terminal.

Even though I was glad to leave the hospital after being away from home for two weeks, I dreaded going home. At least the hospital was safe and other people were involved with Ray and me. We were going home to wait, for what I wasn't sure. But I knew that at this stage Ray would not have found much value in his life. I didn't know if I could handle being witness to this for much longer and was terribly frightened of the tomorrows that were yet unknown to us.

When I got to Ray's room, he was angry. As soon as I entered the room, I saw a look of disgust on his face that I'm not sure I had ever seen before. He began to rant about not trusting me, telling me that I had let him down. He said that he trusted the employees (those in the hospital, I imagine) more than he trusted me. I kept asking him how I had let him down, but he repeated the same thing over and over again. "I can't trust you. I trust the employees more than you." He went on and on; my already tenuous composure faded. I couldn't stand it any longer. I was hurting so badly and this just compounded the pain. I needed someone to help me, but instead tried to calm myself and Ray by putting my arms around him. He did not respond.

The nurses came in to get Ray ready to leave. I went out into the hall and felt my insides open. It was a tormenting, anguished pain that could not be soothed. Everything within me cried out for this to stop. "God help me. Don't do this to us. Please help us." But the reality that two weeks of discovery had imposed upon me was finally crashing down on me in the hall outside Ray's room.

ELEVEN

Ray had been home from the hospital for ten days. His pace-maker had been working well, and we had transmitted our first EKG over the phone to Duke. But Ray was eating poorly, generally only one meal a day. He was also having more and more trouble with showering and shaving. We now had to adjust the water temperature, hand him the soap, put shampoo on his hair, and hand him a towel. He still was able to get in and out of the shower and wash himself fairly well.

There seemed to be more periods in which Ray was quite impatient. One day he said something that I didn't hear because I was in a different room. I asked him to repeat it (perhaps twice) when he said, "I told you ten times already." Then he repeated the statement, loudly enunciating each syllable. I had never seen him behave that way before.

He also wanted one of us home all the time, and needed to know exactly where we were. One night when Ray went up to the bedroom, I stayed down in the den. A few minutes later he angrily called for me and said that I was always disappearing and abandoning him.

Marjorie Leigh, the doctor I had met through the Alzheimer's support group, and her fiancé Stu invited us over for dinner one Sunday afternoon. Ray and I rarely went out. I was careful to try to choose low-risk environments. I was torn about going, but thought we'd give it a try. Marjorie and Stu were well aware of Ray's limitations. If they were game, I would be, too.

The dinner was difficult for me. Ray was quiet; he waited for me to cut his meat, but seemed to manage pretty well otherwise by himself. He did not participate in any of the conversation; I was extremely uncomfortable.

After dinner Stu asked Ray if he'd like to throw the frisbee.

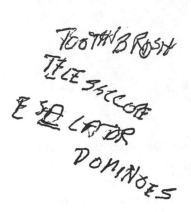

Though Ray could spell these
words orally, this was the
result when he attempted to
write them down.

Ray said he would, but as soon as he tried he was acutely aware
that he could no longer throw or catch. Surprisingly, he remembered that a year before, in California, when we had visited
Warren and Goldie on our way to Hawaii, he and Warren had
tried to play frisbee on the beach. Even then Ray had great
trouble, and Warren had commented on how out of shape he
seemed to be.

August 3

I don't know what it means, but Ray seems more alert. His
memory seems improved and he has had almost no difficulty
with the bathroom for the past few days. We went to see *War
Games*, and Ray seemed able to follow the story line. He has
answered the telephone and remembered who called.

But all is not well. He remembered our friends, the Browns,
are coming to visit from Rhode Island and asked me when they
were coming. When I said they were coming next week, he said
that I was either lying or postponing it.

I registered the power of attorney the other day so that I can
begin to take assets out of Ray's name. It has been emotionally
difficult to do, but if at some point Ray needs to be placed in a
nursing home, it might be best if he has no assets. In that way
our life savings may not have to be spent on nursing home care.

I hate doing it, but I tell myself that it doesn't change a thing between us, or what I feel about him. I will make sure he is cared for.

But by the middle of August the alertness that had been noticeable to others, as well as myself, disappeared. It seemed to happen suddenly. Ray took a nap one evening and when he woke up he could not speak. His inability to speak lasted about forty minutes. The next night he was up and wandered all night. Within a week we saw further deterioration.

Watching TV one day Ray heard a character say, "Then I went inside the light." Ray commented, "Now there's a guy who's having problems!" He laughed, and so did I.

Ray was becoming more and more incontinent and relieved himself anywhere if we weren't there to help him; one day in a basket of dried flowers, another time in a bathroom drawer, but mostly on the floor or carpet. It had become a major problem. I had contacted a carpet cleaning service and they had recommended a product that was used to clean animal urine. The kids and I had become experts in how to absorb and clean urine from carpets. I had ordered so much of the product that I thought I should at least have some stock in the company.

I knew that incontinence pants were available from a variety of sources, but I just couldn't bring myself to have Ray use them. I knew that would come, but it seemed demeaning to put "diapers" (as people in our Alzheimer's group called them) on Ray, who was sometimes surprisingly aware. I had found, that in any change I made, I had to have the reality brutally forced on me before I was ready to take the necessary step.

I had waited too long to get help in the house for Ray. I had waited too long before I made him stop driving or stop smoking. But to take away a person's dignity . . . I knew the day would come when I could no longer put this off either. But, for now, we would try to anticipate and avoid problems.

By the end of August we had a renter in our downstairs apartment: a nice young man who was a student in the Physician's Assistant program at Bowman Gray School of Medicine. He was to be married in December, and at that time his wife would join him.

School started before Labor Day, and Adam came to work full-time. I never knew what I would find when I got home from school each day. One afternoon I came home to find David up in our bedroom with Ray. When David and Ray came downstairs, David told me that he had arrived home from school about four to find Ray and Adam outside. One of the car doors was open. Ray had the car keys in his hand. He was wearing a new shirt of David's, but he had it on backwards. He had one shoe on one foot, and two socks on the other with no shoe. David had told Adam that he could leave, and then he took Ray in to dress him. He was angry that Ray was allowed to go out that way. It reinforced how dependent and vulnerable Ray was. Without someone to make decisions for him, he could look like a witless fool.

August 27

Last night Ray wandered most of the night. This morning I found the refrigerator door open. It must have been open for a good part of the night. I have tried to figure out a way to keep Ray from opening it during the night. I have tied the handles together, but so far, have not figured out anything that works.

At the parcourse this morning I wore my headset, listened to music, and cried most of the time. As I was leaving I saw a neighbor of ours. I have seen him before at the parcourse and every time I have run into him, I've been crying. I was really embarrassed. He must think that this is all I do. Sometimes I think it is.

I think about Ray's dying. I've done that before and believe that when we fantasize about things, it is a way of preparing. I think I have done that a lot in my life, and I believe it helps, so I don't fight those images as much. Sometimes I wish that God would take him. It frightens me to think of what it would be like. But, at the same time, I don't know how I can watch much longer.

My friend Jan came over one afternoon soon after school started. She hadn't seen Ray since we had come back from Duke. She was an understanding friend, always there to listen, able to sense just what to do and say. She had come to know me, the boys, and Ray. She stayed a couple of hours; Ray was in a very confused state. Seeing Ray now must have touched her deeply. We went out on the porch, and she started to cry. We put our arms out and held each other. We didn't have to say anything.

September 6

I am so torn lately. There are times that I feel so distant from Ray. I hardly try and talk with him about anything. I feel that he has become such a burden, that he is keeping me from having a life. I sometimes wish that it were over, but am afraid of what that really means. At other times I reach out to him, stroke his thinning hands and arms, cry, and tell him how much I love him, begging him to come back to me, knowing all the time that it is hopeless. I am always good to him, gentle and caring, but sometimes it wears me down. I feel like I'm in limbo. I can't look ahead, but it's too painful to stay where I am. I try to let go and can't. I grieve so.

This evening Ray stood up and walked behind the chair in which I was sitting. I took his arms and put them around me, stroking him with my cheek and hair, wishing I could bury myself in his once-protective arms. I wanted and needed him. I know it is over, and yet he is there to remind me of what is no longer.

September 8

About 3 : 30 this morning Ray got up and started wandering. He was unable to speak. He pronounced nonsense syllables; repeated them over and over for about ten to fifteen minutes. Intelligible words and phrases were interspersed among the gibberish. In time normal speech returned.

After a short time with Ray, I would start to feel the emptiness of our lives. He was almost oblivious to what was going on. Yet, there remained signs of alertness and pockets of memory. One day, for example, David went to hear philosopher and educator Mortimer Adler speak at Wake Forest University. Ray volunteered a few sentences about him, noting that he was a philosopher. If that isolated incident were looked at out of the context of the rest of Ray's life, one never would have thought that Ray was anything but a normal, functioning man.

David came home from school one day and then left to go to the mall. Ray had seen him leave and went out to go with him. David walked Ray back into the house twice, but after David had left, Ray went out again and waited. He must have been out there for about an hour. Adam was inside watching him because Ray got upset if he thought Adam was hovering. I got home from shopping and asked Ray if he could carry something in for me. He said, "Yes," but instead opened the back door of the car and got in. Adam and I took the groceries in. I tried to get Ray to come out, but he closed the door. It was hot, the windows were closed, but he didn't know where he was.

Finally, I opened the door and told him I'd help him, taking one of his legs and then the other. Then I took his hands and helped him up. Ray hated the heat, but because he was so disoriented, he had aimlessly wandered into the car and did not know what to do. I don't know how long he would have stayed there, if he had been left alone.

My fears of what I might find when I got home from school were sometimes realized. One afternoon in the middle of September, I turned onto our block and saw Adam standing across the street from our house. I wondered why he was there until I got a little bit closer and saw Ray standing in the neighbor's yard dressed only in his underwear. I pulled into the drive and crossed the street to get him. I wasn't sure if I should laugh or cry. I found I wasn't really that upset and joked with Ray that he'd get arrested. "They won't arrest me," he answered. "I won't let them."

Adam was more upset than either Ray or I. He really felt he had failed. Ray had decided to leave the house, and Adam had been unable to stop him. All Adam found he could do was follow Ray and stay with him. I explained to Adam some of the approaches he might have tried, and he said he would do better in the future.

After Adam left, I dressed Ray. As I helped him put on his pants, he told me that they were not his. Then he said I was not putting his socks on right. Later he asked me to get his shoes and socks, even though he was wearing them. He was confused the rest of that afternoon and night.

At dinner he had difficulty picking up his food. He would put the fork under the rim of the plate. When he would finally get the food on a fork (or when I'd put it on a fork for him), he would have difficulty directing it to his mouth.

Around one o'clock the next morning I woke up. Ray was not in bed and I couldn't find him in the kitchen. After looking through the house, I found him in Michael's room with the door closed. He said he was trying to feel his way around. He was not panicked, as he had been at other times when he been "trapped" in a dark room. Things were strewn on the floor and when I found him, he was holding some papers.

September 14

RAY: I'm talking about a pair. That's what I'm talking about!

ME: What pair?

RAY: Any pair! [He was enunciating each word and sounded quite frustrated.] A pair of trousers.

ME: What about them?

RAY: Do they come in pairs or not?

ME: No, trousers don't come in pairs.

RAY: Yes, they do! [Long pause.] How do they come?

ME: They come all ready to wear.

RAY: [Confused. Pause.] As what? You never answered that. As what? A *pair*!

ME: Yes, a pair. But you call them, "one pair." It's just one pant.

RAY: I don't understand.

ME: What part don't you understand?

RAY: All of it. Every single bit of it. The whole category is something I don't understand. Don't you understand how hard it is for me to understand?

ME: I'm trying to.

RAY: It's a big mystery to me, the whole area. And you don't understand that I don't understand the whole thing.

ME: Can you ask me a question?

RAY: Yes! What the hell is this pants all about? Don't you understand that I don't understand any of it? It's a big area that's gone, that's not even there. There's a whole thing out there called pants, that I don't know anything about. Why can't you understand that? . . . I don't know what's so difficult . . . It's as if the earth just opened up and dropped out and you just—'Oh, it's gone. I'll accept it. It's okay.'

ME: No, I'm not saying that.

RAY: I can accept that. There's this big area called pants that I don't understand anything about called pants . . . You don't understand that I don't understand any of it?

ME: Yes, but I don't know where to begin to help you understand it.

RAY: There's a category of things that I don't know anything about. It's just floating in the air.

ME: Can you ask a question about it?

RAY: What is it?

September 23

I woke up at four this morning to Ray's telling me that my head was on upside down. I was in a dead sleep. It's hard enough responding to such a remark when I'm awake, so I'm not sure of exactly what I said. But I do remember Ray's asking me how he could fix the scene. I told him to just turn it around. He said he couldn't. He seemed confused, but not really frightened. About 7 A.M. he awoke and I asked him if things were still upside down. He said, "No." Maybe he didn't even remember what had happened.

School had become a safe haven in my life. I found I was able to function fairly well. I had to leave the tears, pain, fear at the door each day, and as the day progressed, I was usually able to involve myself with the kids and my work.

But there were days that I did not do well, and whenever I had a few moments alone it was as if I could release some of what stayed so locked up in me. Sometimes I wanted someone to say, "What's wrong?" so that I could pour out my heart. What I was feeling was a desperate aloneness and fear for what awaited me.

But I had continual fights with myself. They would start with my experiencing the grief that would overcome me so often. Then I would hear myself saying, "You're not losing Ray, you've lost him already. He wanders around the house not knowing what to do, lost in his own environment. His thoughts are not related to you and he will never be able to give you anything again. You must accept that. You must begin a new life now. You can't wait. Don't think of this as a waiting period, because all you do is hope you'll wake up from the nightmare and that things will be okay. Well, you're not going to wake up and have it okay. The reality is that Ray is demented. He no longer is, and never will be, the person you knew and loved. That pain tears you apart, but that's the reality. No one is going to hand you Ray or a new life. You'll have to do it. Consciously. Purposely. Cry if you must, but do not wallow in self-pity. It will only destroy you."

September 29

I was writing in my journal this morning. Ray was wandering around the house saying, "How can I do that? . . . must find a way to make this continue. It'll be all right." I would have asked him what the problem was, but I knew he wouldn't know.

Reading last night, I came across the word "xenophobia." I didn't know the meaning and thought I'd try Ray who, despite so much loss, still retained a rich vocabulary. "Fear of foreigners," he responded without hesitation.

Since the day I found Ray standing outside in his underwear, I come down our block with eagle-eyes. This afternoon I saw

Adam standing in the driveway two doors away from our house. I pulled the car into our drive and walked over to see what was happening. I had not seen Ray. When I got over to the side of the house, I saw Ray standing in some bushes. He had walked up some brick steps into the bushes and didn't know how to get out. Adam said he had been standing there for about an hour. He thought he was at our house and was angry at Adam, who had tried his best to coax Ray out. When Ray saw me, he became verbally abusive to Adam, who had done nothing to provoke such an attack. "Adam is not obedient. He tries to run my life . . ." He went on and on, but came out of the bushes and back to our house.

I am sorry Adam had to experience such an attack, but he said he understood. I think he did. Adam shared some other incidents that had happened in the past few days. Ray had tried to climb over a split-rail fence between our house and our neighbors', and one afternoon walked down the street, but would not permit Adam to walk with him.

I knew things were getting too difficult for Adam to handle. He was trying very hard, but was not able to cope with the problems that Ray presented. He lacked confidence and found it difficult to assert himself with Ray. Consequently, Ray was placed in precarious and sometimes potentially hazardous situations. It was difficult for Adam to understand how dependent Ray was on him for the simplest of decisions. But despite Ray's lack of judgment and reasoning, he knew that he could not depend on Adam to make those decisions.

I would have to do something else. I had considered adult day care briefly, but didn't think I could stand seeing Ray with people twenty to thirty years older than himself. At forty-seven he looked younger than his years, and it disturbed me that he functioned worse than many people with whom he would come into contact. Besides, I was sure I would never be able to get him up, dressed, and at a center before work. The alternative was to look for more experienced help.

Even though I spent most of my nonworking time at home

with Ray, I found that I was getting out of the house more. I would meet friends for dinner mostly, and I no longer had such terrible feelings about "abandoning" Ray. As long as I knew he was in good hands, especially David's and Michael's (when Michael was home from school), I could leave. Sometimes friends would stay with Ray, and—although I always worried that there might be a problem, especially with the bathroom— David and I welcomed the respite. I was truly learning that we are our brother's keeper. I just hoped that I could give to others what they were giving to me.

October 4

Ray is almost always confused and it is rare that he expresses a series of sensible thoughts. Last night he kept asking if the seams were straight when we were in bed and if it was even. I don't know what he really meant, but he often talks about things being out of sync, "not meshing, not right." When he's in bed he often asks me, "Am I straight? Is this right?" It seems to be an attempt to organize the confusion and chaos that he is experiencing.

I found someone new to help care for Ray. I hated to tell Adam because he has come to care for and about Ray. He is a gentle and caring man who I am sure will be able to help someone else. But Ray needs someone with whom he can feel more confident.

After deciding I needed to find another caregiver for Ray, I wrote to about fifteen churches in town explaining our need. The day after I sent out the letters, a man called me. He introduced himself as Ben Brimson. He told me that his minister had received my letter and contacted him. We talked briefly on the phone, and then Ben came out to meet us.

He was a sixty-five-year-old retiree who had lived and worked in the area his entire life. He spoke with a rural Southern accent and seemed to shuffle his words together. I had to listen carefully to make sure I understood everything he said. He lived with his wife and one daughter who was about to graduate from high school. He had another daughter, who was married, and one grandchild.

Among other jobs, Ben had been the meat cutter and stockroom manager for one of the K&W Cafeterias in Winston. He had also spent a number of years delivering milk, and stayed in touch with many of his old customers. He had slipped and fallen at work one day about two years earlier while carrying 150 pounds of meat. He was left with an obvious limp.

He told me that as a young man he had been tall and gangly. Now his jowls were full and his shirts bulged around his middle. But his eyes sparkled. From the beginning I found Ben to be genuinely in love with life and people. He embraced those he met with his natural, uncomplicated humility and his warm, jovial manner. If any hurt or personal pain existed in Ben's heart, it never showed. He was always the same: steady, dependable, caring.

Ben had been raised on a small dairy farm in rural North Carolina. His father had died when he was two, and by the time he entered school, he was milking six or seven cows a day as well as handling the plow. He proudly told me of the time his picture had appeared in the *Progressive Farmer*, a rural magazine, in 1930, when he was twelve. He had produced one of the largest wheat crops in his county.

Ben's church was an integral part of his life; he lived his religion. He seemed to reach out to everyone and set no man apart. He not only fulfilled our needs, but he gave unstintingly of himself to others. He had cared for a friend of his who had recently died and continued to spend time with the man's adult daughter, who was a victim of cerebral palsy. Even before he retired, Ben would go to his friend's house on his lunch hour and after work to help the young woman with tasks she could not manage herself.

What Ben seemed to like most was talking and telling jokes, never seeming to tire of them or remember that I had heard them before. But he was also quiet—sensitive and responsive to Ray's needs and able to handle the times when Ray became confused and agitated. Without cajoling or acting overly solicitous, with patience and consideration, he assisted with the tasks that for Ray were impossible to face alone.

There was something kind and gentle about this big man who sat with us that afternoon. I could tell from the beginning that he would value and respect Ray regardless of how he functioned. I cannot recall a single instance when Ben talked about Ray in front of him, even though it was clear that Ray rarely understood. Ben was good-natured and responsive to Ray's needs, and I grew to know what his minister meant when he said, "I think God retired Ben so that he could help others."

October 9

Ray was up about one this morning, walking around the house. In the bedroom (he thought he was in the living room) he kept trying to put things in different places. He used his hands to point and explain, talking about straight lines, curves, one thing moving to another place. He wanted me to move things, pointing to an empty space, the blanket, or a sweater. When I said I couldn't, he said then he would have to. I did not understand one thing he was trying to explain, but he was very serious. He knew I didn't understand, but he kept trying to explain so that I would. How frustrated he must have been!

Late that afternoon Ray talked about things being filled or empty and about reflections. Again, I didn't know what he was talking about.

"You're being deliberately obtuse. Don't be so dumb. I hate when you're dumb," he said in an accusing tone.

In bed that night to himself: "We should peel back the other sheet and make room in the bed. Right? Okay, let's make our stuff ready. Where are we coming from here? Are we going to be ready? Let's get ourselves ready for this. We should be ready for this half. We should be ready for this piece and the other piece. We have to fit ourselves in. Here, this piece will accept us. [He was holding up a part of the blanket.] What are you writing?"

I told him I was trying to record the things he said.

He laughed a little. He did not seem to mind. Instead, he seemed pleased, as if what he was saying was important enough to record.

"This will fit you," he continued. "You could fold this into half of it. Half of it will be left over in the other half. It will fit. Know what I mean? This will apparently fit into half of it. Know what I mean?"

In bed about three the next morning: "My chests are uneven. My sides are uneven." I asked him what he meant. "If you measure them they're not the same. You can't divide them evenly in half."

Later that day: "Three and two—odd and even. We have to accommodate ourselves to odd and even."

I read some of the conversations quoted above to Michael and David that day. Ray commented, "I sure do give good advice."

So much of Ray's expressive language had to do with organization, putting things together, making parts and pieces fit. Was it an attempt to organize his crumbling world? It was as if things had become so fragmented for him that he was struggling to put it in some kind of order. Were his perceptions so distorted that he truly saw and experienced that which he attempted to make clear to me? What was it like for him? Would I ever really know?

TWELVE

Sometimes I wondered if I would survive emotionally, mentally, or financially. How many more months or years would we have to endure this slow destruction? In the fall of 1983, I wrote an opinion piece for the *Winston-Salem Sentinel* in which I attempted to describe some of the problems faced by families of Alzheimer's victims and sufferers of other dementias:

. . . I find that there are no insurance programs or public funds to assist with custodial or personal-needs care. Skilled nursing care is a coverage provided by most insurance policies as well as Medicare, but there are no provisions for those requiring personal-needs care in or out of an institutional setting. Consequently, I must shoulder the financial responsibility for perhaps years of care alone . . . The disease of the century? A silent epidemic? Perhaps. Certainly, it's an increasing problem of major proportions for public and often personal concern. What is needed is an expanded definition of skilled nursing care to include, rather than exclude, those who have personal-needs care. Those in our society in need of supervision and management because of impaired functions may require different, but no less care than those in need of skilled nursing services. Insurance plans and public programs must examine provisions which exclude those in need of personal-needs care. To me, such provisions are discriminatory and unjust, leaving families with no financial support. Although Medicaid pays for personal-needs care in many states, an individual must be a pauper to qualify . . .

Because of the insurance coverage we had, Ray's *medical* expenses were reimbursed—except for about $500. All told, Ray was hospitalized for ten weeks, at a total cost of about $60,000.

But more worrisome was home and nursing care. Adam and Ben both worked for very little. For the eight months that I employed one or the other of them, I paid approximately $3,500. I was very fortunate, however; far more typical is $35 for an eight-hour shift. Care in a nursing home in our area costs

$18,000 to $24,000 a year—much more in other parts of the country—and the cost is increasing every year. Medicaid will pay for nursing care—if the patient and his family have no assets. Others must "spend down," ridding themselves of everything they have, before they qualify.

October 13

Ray wrote a note to David that I could not read. I asked him to read it to me. He read: "Dear David, I want you to know that I love you very much. Your daddy."

October 15

Watching a TV game show today, Ray saw a contestant being shown a BMW and a Chevrolet logo. Ray identified them immediately.

Watching *All's Quiet on the Western Front*, Ray remembered the name of Corporal Himmelstoss. He also remarked, "There's a moving scene in the film with men singing before they go off to war."

October 17

I have been looking for the thermostat cover for a few days. I found it today in the dryer. Ray had taken it off and put it in his pants pocket.

Ray "opened" a glass today. He turned it upside down and used a church key. The glass broke. He was not hurt and unaware of what had happened.

October 18

RAY: There's all kinds of rules to things and I just don't know how to do it.

ME: Rules for what things?

RAY: Anything that has to be together; that has to go together . . . Like . . . umm . . . all the crystals have to be a certain color. They have to match. You have to work with crystals a certain way. They all have to string together—with rules.

Ray's moments of clarity were among the most painful parts of this time. One evening he told me he thought his brain was damaged. He could not elaborate or seem to be able to attach much feeling to that thought, but he knew. I told him we would always be with him—that he would never be alone and that he needed to try to feel safe in knowing that.

October 20

Our support group is planning an Information Night for interested members of the community to learn about Alzheimer's disease and related disorders. Making a flyer that we plan to distribute announcing the meeting reminded me of Ray sitting at his drawing board. He used to use the same kind of press type that I used. I had watched him often. How I loved seeing him work. His shirtsleeves rolled up to his elbows, his face concentrating intently on perfecting what he was drawing. How much pride he took in what he produced. How in love I was with those hands that were so talented, that held me, that made me feel so protected and loved.

Even now, at those rare times when he returns a hug, I melt remembering . . . I don't want to forget, but the memories hurt so much.

Last night about 3 A.M. I woke to find Ray out of bed. I called and heard his voice. I found him in David's room with the door almost closed. I pushed it a little and felt it stop. Ray was curled up, lying on the floor behind the door. He had gone into the bedroom, voided, and lay down on the floor. "Let's go to bed, Honey," I said. He got up and came willingly. When I got him into bed and tucked him in, he said, "Boy this is a comfortable bed." He was like a little confused child and my heart broke. I held him and cried. We both fell asleep.

In late October Ray lost bowel control for the first time since the disastrous incident in the hospital. It wasn't really that he physically couldn't control it; it was as though the memory of how and what to do were not there. I hoped, unrealistically, that it wouldn't happen again.

October 31

Ray began a conversation this evening by saying, "I should really have asked whatever I wanted for the next person in line. It was wasted on me." I asked him what was wasted on him. He told me, "Anything I wanted."

The conversation went back and forth with Ray repeating the same thing over and over. When I asked him what he felt he had accomplished, he said, "Nothing. I accomplished no ambition because I was entitled to no ambition." He continued by denying that he had ever had a successful career or even ever worked.

"Didn't you make money and support all of us?" I asked. He answered, "I never earned any amount of support, in terms of any just amount. I earned zero. That's what I earned—zero."

When I told him that he worked at Design, Inc. and had earned a lot of money in his life he answered, "I wasn't entitled to any money."

"Why not? You worked hard. You were talented."

"I was not."

"Yes, you were, Honey. Think of all the things you were able to do."

"Like what?"

"You drew so well. You designed so well."

"That's true. There was never any sum of money."

"You were paid for that, though. You remember you had Colony as a project at Design, Inc.?"

"Uh-huh."

"Do you remember what you did on that job?"

"I don't know what I did on that job."

Sometimes Ben took Ray out to watch a neighborhood ball game or for an ice-cream soda. As they entered the house one afternoon, Ray asked, "Who lives here?"

One evening Ray said, "Do you know who I miss? I miss my father. Ben is taking the place of my father." When I asked him

Asked to reconstruct this message, Ray said he had written that he wanted to go shopping and eat Chinese food. The figure at upper right is intended to be $10.

if he knew where his father was, he said he didn't. I asked him if he knew about his mother. He didn't remember that either. I told him that both his parents had died. He looked surprised and wanted to know how I could know that. He said, "I'll have to call my sisters and check on that."

Watching a TV show about lottery winners, Ray asked, "Did we win? Are we rich?"

Always trying to see what memory Ray still had and how oriented he was, I asked him one day what state he lived in. He answered, "State of confusion."

Ray saw Robert McNamara on television. He told me that he was one of "Ford's whiz kids," but later did not recognize Michael and David in a photograph I showed him.

Watching a TV commercial one day, Ray asked, "Under what circumstances will he sell those bulbs? Can I buy a dozen? Ten? How much? Is he going to sell any? Can't I find out? Will he sell me those bulbs?"

December 3

ME: Tell me the riddle you told me you solved.
RAY: What riddle?
ME: About the black man—about substituting a black man. Do you remember what you said?
RAY: No.
ME: You said you can substitute a black man for a french fry.
RAY: [Laughing.] I said that? What was I talking about?

ME: That doesn't make sense?

RAY: No. [Laughing while talking.] A black man for a french fry?

ME: That's what you said a few minutes ago.

RAY: That's too complicated. It wasn't a free substitution. It just doesn't make sense.

December 6

I heard Ray in the middle of the night. He was standing about a foot from the bed, holding on to the light bulb from the reading lamp. He was afraid he was going to fall and held on to the first thing he saw. I stood in front of him and held him around the waist while taking his hand from the bulb. He was very frightened and I had to push him, holding on to his hands to get him to sit down. I've seen him like that before. He becomes practically paralyzed, forgetting the sequence of movements involved in actions such as walking. I guess it's not that different from not knowing how to dress and undress, eat, go to the bathroom, get from one room to another. Sometimes he can't remember how to begin, and at other times he loses the memory in the middle of a task and can't continue.

Early in December I went to San Diego to visit Warren and Goldie for a few days. Michael would be home to help David for the weekend, and Ben would be there during the weekdays. I felt that they would manage fine. Before I left, Ray told me that I should eat out for him when I was in California. I asked him where? What kind of food? He told me Chinese. I didn't know how aware he was of what he was saying, but it made it easier to go. I had come to the point where I knew that Ray could not be with me, that we could no longer enjoy life together, and that as lonely as it was, it was not forsaking him for me to do things without him.

December 10

Sitting on the plane reminded me of the last time I was on a plane. It was our trip to Hawaii almost a year and a half ago. I remember how I held on to Ray. I must have known someplace within me even then that I was losing him. He was different and I was scared. I had told Warren and Goldie [when we had stopped off in California] that something was wrong with him, but at the time was angry. I thought it was within Ray's power to control it, or at least try. But he was so apathetic, didn't seem to care.

I will not miss the Ray I am losing now. He needs and depends on me, but there is only a past between us. I miss the old Ray. The Ray that would devour new things to learn, new places to explore. The Ray who enjoyed life and looked forward to the future, who delighted in pleasing his kids and me. I miss him and if he were home, I would want to be with him. But the Ray at home is someone I don't know. The boys will take care of him and, although he will ask for me, it won't be the same.

Goldie was late picking me up at the airport and while I waited, I remembered. The flashes of memories, and there are so many, swoop over me and seem to wash my soul like warm running water. But they pierce and sting too.

I remember how Ray and I used to greet each other at the airport when he would come to Detroit to visit me or I would go to New York. How strange and awkward it was at first. We had known each other such a short time, just meeting at camp in June and knowing by the end of the summer that we would marry.

I had gone back to Brooklyn after camp and stayed with his family a few days before going back to school. Then Ray had come to Detroit for a few days in September, again in October, and brought me an engagement ring in November at Thanksgiving.

We had been in the kitchen late Thanksgiving eve when he handed me a ring box. I opened it to find a small ring with something shiny at the top about the size of a pin top. I didn't know anything about jewelry, but I had never seen a ring quite so pathetic. Before I could respond, Ray took a velvet blue ring box out of his pocket and said, "Maybe you'd like this better."

Inside was a lovely diamond engagement ring. I really hadn't expected one and didn't think it mattered if I had one or not. But wearing it made me feel so special. I was so conscious of it and felt it was a way of broadcasting my happiness. Ray had returned to New York, but the ring was there for me until we could be together again.

I wanted to have a good time in San Diego. I wanted to get away so that I could cope better when I went home. But the memories kept creeping into my consciousness. I couldn't let go.

Goldie and I sat and talked in the hot tub for most of the afternoon. As always, I found it easy to tell her how I really felt. In the evening we drove to Mexico with some friends of theirs. For the first time I was the "extra," the "odd number," the one who was alone. I tried to shake the feeling, telling myself we were just five people going to dinner together. But I knew that wasn't true. I tried to participate in the conversations, but I was constantly on the verge of tears. They were all very nice to me and tried to include me, but I continued to feel alone. They belonged to each other, and I was by myself. I knew I was indulging in an enormous amount of self-pity, but couldn't seem to free myself of it. I just wanted to go home. I just wanted to cry.

I found the evening a disaster. I spent most of the time fighting the tears that forced their way to the surface, waiting to be released. In the car on the way home, it was dark, and I could no longer fight back my feelings. I had become quite adept at crying silently with Ray. Often in bed I would cry and not want Ray to know. So I had learned to let the tears come without making a sound or movement. Before we got to the border we stopped to buy some Kahlua. Everyone got out of the car except Goldie and me. She must have known, even though I was doing my best to control myself. All that pent-up hurt I had been holding for hours poured out. She just held me, and it helped.

I did better after that. One evening we went to a birthday party with lots of Warren and Goldie's friends. Another day we visited Sea World, and then went on to Fat's City, a 1930s art deco bar and restaurant for a happy hour which turned into dinner. Before I left we went to Seaport Village where we walked, talked, looked around the shops, and ended up at a pleasant Mexican restaurant for lunch.

Aside from the first night, my trip to San Diego helped. Each step was painful. But I left knowing I would make it. Somehow I would come to know how to balance memories with a new life. I would have to.

December 18

I often have this image of two amorphous creatures running along a path. The first one wears a sign on his back that says "Intellect." The second wears a sign that reads "Emotion." Intellect runs along the path at a comfortable pace, breathing easy, confident about the outcome, clearly focused. But Emotion struggles desperately. He can see Intellect ahead of him, wants to run even with him, but fights to just narrow the distance. There are times he catches Intellect, running even for a while. But it is not long before Intellect gets a burst of energy, runs ahead again, and Emotion loses ground.

That is often the struggle I am in. I find that I understand what is happening intellectually long before I can accept and be relatively at ease with it emotionally. I just hope that Emotion isn't a loser. I hope he eventually catches up and can run comfortably next to Intellect. I am really rooting for him.

December 20

I think Ray has taken another dip. The other night he wet the bed for the first time, other than in the hospital. He was unaware that he had. In addition, for the past few days, Ray has been unable to anticipate that he has to use the bathroom. Often our only signal from him is when he starts to "dance" like a child who has waited until the last minute.

He is slower, quieter, and appears more disoriented. He has more difficulty identifying people in pictures, more difficulty eating, doesn't ask to go anywhere, and is becoming afraid of the stairs.

December 24

Today was a special day—very happy and terribly sad. I vacillated between feeling content and sad all day, sometimes feeling
both simultaneously. This evening we all worked together to
get what has become a traditional Christmas Eve fondue dinner
ready. We made onion soup with gobs of mozzarella cheese
melted on top, cubed pieces of beef and chicken, prepared four
or five different sauces, and tossed a salad. Wonderful neighbors
brought us all kinds of Christmas goodies, some of which we
added to our table. We turned on some music and the scene
was set.

We sat down at our festive table, the kids talking about past
Christmas vacations, skiing this winter, how slowly the meat
always seems to cook, and why it is best to have two skewers
going at the same time. We are rarely together anymore. Michael
off at school; David frequently off at dinner because he has a
job at McDonald's. It is often just Ray and me for dinner. Dinners that are silent. Dinners where I cut up Ray's food, often
have to start him, or even feed him. But tonight was different,
and I soaked up the warmth and love that filled our home, hoping that Ray could, in spite of his inability to verbalize, also experience it.

I knew I was being corny, and the kids would probably say,
"Oh, Mom!" But I took a chance. "Could we all join hands?" I
asked, "and each share how we're feeling about being together?" There wasn't any, "Oh, Mom," as I had expected. Instead David and Michael each took one of Ray's hands, and I
took Michael's and David's.

David went first and said, "I love you all." Ray was next and
repeated what David had just said. Michael said, "I could never
hope for a better family in the whole world." It was my turn
and I said, "If I had my life to live over again I'd choose to be
with all of you, even knowing what I know now." There were
tears in my eyes and I know there were tears in my brave boys'
hearts.

Later in the evening Ray was in the den with Michael. I could hear Michael repeatedly asking him if he was okay. He took Ray to the bathroom and then helped him lie down in bed. Michael came downstairs and the three of us sat at the kitchen table. I think it was the first time that the three of us sat and talked about Ray's getting worse and dying; about if we wanted, or if he would want, to prolong his life by intervening, should that decision have to be made.

David said little, and later I noticed that he was not around. I found him crying in his bedroom. "I love you so much," he told me as I stroked and talked to him while he continued to sob. I told him how good he was and how lucky Daddy was to have him. He was lucky to have a daddy like Ray, too, and that he would have wonderful memories. He would be a special person and father to his own children because of his relationship with Ray.

David came downstairs later, and the boys and Ray watched skiing on TV, reminiscing about ski trips we had taken. Ray said he remembered whatever the kids asked him about, but when they pursued it with other questions, it was clear that he didn't remember.

Ray really is like a dying man lately. He can barely do much more than stand and sit. He has not participated in any conversation in the last week and is unable to decide on anything, including knowing if he has to use the bathroom, or what he wants to drink.

By early January Ray was wetting the bed at night, and I purchased some additional rubber sheets. He would not know he had wet, but would awaken soaked and uncomfortable, unable to resolve his problem. I would get him up, change his underwear, change the bedding, and tuck him back in. It was like having a child.

Ray was almost nonverbal and also appeared depressed. He seemed to know something was terribly wrong, but did not know what. If I asked him what was the matter, he would say, "I don't know."

With Michael back at school, showering and shaving became monumental chores for David and me. We had reduced showering to once a week on Saturdays, and we both dreaded it. Ray became verbally abusive and would scream that we were killing him. David had been fairly successful at distracting him by talking about football, TV, or what he was going to wear, but even that didn't work very often anymore. Ray was terrified of getting into the tub and hated the feel of the water.

But even with all our difficulties getting Ray to shave, we never seriously considered having him grow a beard. He had grown one once, years before, and neither of us had liked the way he looked. Letting him grow a beard would have made me feel that I was neglecting him; and I think that keeping Ray clean-shaven was another way of holding on to the Ray I wanted back.

January 4

Yesterday I shaved Ray. We had not shaved him in three days and he looked grubby. I know the longer we wait, the harder it is. I have learned not to ask him if he wants to, but rather just walk him into the bathroom and turn on the shaver, talking as I'm shaving him. Today he was almost in tears. He started to rant, and although he could have pushed me away, did not. He doesn't even know that he has any free will or control. He did push my hand away and tell me he "won't put up with it," but allowed me to continue. At one point he realized that I was trying to distract him with conversation and accused me of treating him like a child. I said that he had to shave, that he couldn't go around unshaven. I tried to assure him that I wouldn't hurt him. I never raised my voice, but just tried to get it over with as quickly as possible.

Afterward, he lay down on the bed. He was still upset. I stroked and kissed him and told him I loved him. I said that I knew that this was very hard for him, that he was the center of my life and I had grown so much because of him. How much he understood, I don't know. I needed to say it anyway. Probably more for me than for him. Always at times like that I think of the old Ray. What would he do or say? It helps for me to know that if it had been me who had become so impaired, he would have done everything necessary, willingly and selflessly.

I knew that somewhere within Ray he was aware that something had robbed him of his dignity, his reasoning, his ability to function. I believe that his frequent depressed moods were due to that awareness, however limited it was. I think he knew on some primitive, instinctive level, like an infant or an animal in pain or distress.

My journal was an assortment of isolated feelings, incidents, and conversations. On New Year's Eve I wrote: "I watched the apple come down on Times Square and cried a little. I cried out of gratitude for the past; hope and fear for the future." I wrote about the loneliness I felt when Marjorie Leigh, who had become a friend, moved to another state. And I made a note about the day I happened to ask Ray if he remembered Rommel's first name. He unhesitatingly answered, "Erwin."

Those responses never ceased to amaze me. So much was gone, and yet there were glimpses of the Ray I once knew— poignant reminders of what was. Though they brought a warm smile to my face, they also produced agonizing pain.

I wrote of the agony Ray experienced in his last months at Design, Inc. and of his futile attempts to understand for how much of what had happened he was responsible. I had contacted Eleanor, his former boss, twice during Ray's initial hospitalization over a year earlier, but she was never to call Ray or me. She never sent a card or contacted us in any way. It was only as Ray became more and more demented that the pain of his days at Design, Inc. subsided. Finally, he just forgot.

But I didn't. I wanted to understand. I even wanted to forgive. I wanted Eleanor to come to me and apologize, not for taking Ray off the job, not for not knowing, but for having hurt him so. I wanted her to contact him and somehow convey that she cared—to tell him how, as students, he had affected her life and how she had benefited from having known him. But she didn't. And I could not forgive.

*   *

I came home from school one afternoon in January and commented to Ray, "You like it when I'm home. I can tell."

"I do," he answered.

"Why?" I asked.

"I feel complete."

"What do you mean 'complete'?"

"Like the missing pieces are filled."

January 20

Ray slept late this morning. When he woke he was in a foul mood. He was kicking the covers and angry, but didn't know why. The dreaded Saturday shower loomed before me, but I felt I could handle it today. As angry and agitated as he gets, he never strikes me. Sometimes he seems close to it, but he doesn't. I walked him into the bathroom. It wasn't until we were in the bathroom and he was undressed that he realized that he was to shower. But I had learned that preparing him was worse. Generally, it was just better to tell him as we were into the activity.

Getting him to lift his foot to get into the tub took a good five minutes. He didn't remember. As usual, he complained bitterly about the water temperature, but he didn't seem to know if it was too hot or too cold. He either doesn't have the concept any longer or cannot attach the word to the meaning.

He literally screamed that I was hurting him and that he was freezing. He gritted his teeth and yelled, "Goddamn you," over and over. He was near tears, and his frustration and helplessness must have overwhelmed him. The further along we got, the more upset he got. He began to scream at me. "I hate you! I hate this! I hate the feel of it!" He was almost crying. "You don't know when to stop! *Stop!* I'm begging you to stop."

I was beginning to break. I wanted to shower him quickly and get him out. We are only showering him once a week. Should I abandon the showers because they are so torturous? "You bitch," he yelled, and I broke. With me crying and Ray screaming and cursing, I got him out of the shower and got him dressed.

He calmed down as he began to feel warmer and more comfortable. David had been asleep, but the tumult woke him. He came into the bedroom and put his arms around me and told me he loved me. Then he drew Ray to us and held us both.

By the beginning of February Ray's hands were shaking. He was not able to lift a cup to his mouth or hold an eating utensil because his hands shook so. He also began to fall. He would attempt to sit down on a chair, but would misjudge the distance and fall next to the chair, instead.

He was losing bowel control more frequently, but I told myself that they were only isolated incidents and I would handle them as they arose. I still couldn't bring myself to use incontinence pants. Handling his bladder and bowel problems was really just a matter of being able to anticipate when he had to use the bathroom and getting him there. But we weren't doing a very good job of being able to anticipate.

Ray was also becoming more negative. Ben saw it during the day and so did we. It was not just when it came to showering and shaving, but it seemed generally more pervasive. Ray was far more demanding as well, unwilling to postpone anything.

I was still going to the parcourse in the morning before work. Martha, a friend and neighbor, and I went each morning. She would listen every day to the events of the past day and night. She provided as much of a release for me as did any exercise we might do. But since David was still asleep when I left, I knew it was really like leaving Ray alone. I would frequently come home to a wet floor somewhere in the house. I was becoming more and more concerned about Ray's safety. With his falling, I knew I was taking a chance. But I hated to give it up.

One afternoon I came home from work and smelled disinfectant. Ray was wearing a different pair of pants than I had put on him in the morning. Without being too graphic, Ben told me that Ray had defecated and there had been a big mess to clean—Ray, carpeting, cushions, clothing. Ben had handled it admirably. In fact, he joked about it, taking it in stride.

After Ben left I saw that, although he had done an excellent job, I would still have to clean the carpet, as well as some cushion covers. I took the covers off the couch and loveseat and went downstairs to put them in the washing machine. When I hit the bottom step, I almost died. The downstairs was a lake. We had had a severe rain that afternoon, and a small hole in the foundation had allowed what seemed like gallons of water to pour in. Water had rushed in and soaked a good part of the downstairs carpet. I couldn't believe it! Upstairs! Downstairs! What next?

It was ten o'clock when I fell into bed that night. The couch and loveseat covers were washed and back where they belonged. I had rented a carpet shampooer and had cleaned the upstairs carpet. Jim, the fellow who lived downstairs, and I had suctioned up all of the water downstairs. I slept well that night, knowing it was time for a long overdue step. My house was going to be destroyed, and Ray was too aware of what was happening to him for me to delude myself that I was saving him from being humiliated.

THIRTEEN

There were mornings when a part of me wished Ray would just not wake up. In the past six months he had become incontinent and begun to lose bowel control; he spent most of his life in a confused state. His hands shook so that he could not eat, even when he could manage the sequence of food to utensil to mouth; he had to be fed almost everything he ate. He could not walk up steps without falling. He could not put an article of clothing on himself, and was often not even able to cooperate by lifting his arm or leg. He spent his life sleeping, sitting, and eating. He could not interact with us, and I felt that all I provided was love, protection, and security. How much he even knew of that, I'm not sure. But I do believe he felt most secure when he was with his family.

I knew I could no longer put off having Ray wear some kind of incontinence pants. It took a minor disaster to make me realize that it was probably worse for him to know that something embarrassing and degrading had occurred than for us to avoid it with appropriate precautions. When I actually put them on, Ray did not seem to care. He never complained about them, but did occasionally refer to them as his "diapers" and questioned why there were so bulky.

In late February he seemed to have periods of awareness. Sometimes he would say he was "disgusted" or "sick of it." When I'd ask him what he was disgusted at or sick of, he would say that he didn't know. He couldn't identify what was so disturbing, but he appeared in terrible mental anguish. He would sometimes ask what was wrong with him or where this would end. He would not have understood or, I think, wanted to hear the answer. So I would just hold him.

Ray's balance got worse. He fell frequently, sometimes hitting his head, and once fell flat on his face because he was unable to put his hands out in front of him to break his fall. Even when we'd hold him, he'd lose his balance, usually on the stairs. He had such a difficult time with the seven steps he had to climb. He would walk into the riser, which acted as a prompt to remind him to lift his leg. When he finally got to the top of the stairs, he would take another step up since he was not able to anticipate a change in the walking pattern. He negotiated the stairs as if he were on a ladder. He'd teeter in all directions, and when he'd lose his balance, would fall. I could barely get him up and to the landing. He was unable to stand by himself, and I would have to lift him one step at a time. He was so helpless, but he allowed me to pull and drag him up those few steps. He'd be exhausted, as I was, after the ordeal.

Ray had become more passive than ever. He did not wander much at night anymore, and would often sit in a chair for an entire day. David was working, which meant that there was less time for him to help with Ray. Friends volunteered to stay so that I could get out in the evening. I felt able to call on friends for emergencies, but not to go to a movie or shopping, or to just get out.

Ray had spent the past year and a half relatively unaware of what was happening to him. But one day in March, he became very upset. He had had times when he seemed to know that something was happening, but those times were fleeting and his awareness was usually such that he was not able to attach the intellectual understanding to appropriate emotions. But on this day, it was different. He kept repeating that he was sick and asked me what was wrong with him, what would happen to him. He knew something was terribly wrong but couldn't identify or verbalize what, and I believe even if I had told him, he would not have comprehended. He was in terrible mental anguish.

March 1

I told Ray in bed last night that he has been the most significant person in my life and I hoped he would always know that.

As I held back my never-ending supply of tears, I asked him how that made him feel. He said, "Wonderful."

March 10

. . . And the future. Will I know how bad it is? Do I really even know now? Will I know when I can't handle it anymore? I see it. I know it. And part of me believes it. But I want to scream, "Damn you! Damn you! You are taking this precious, precious part of my life! Don't let it be! I need him! I want him! Damn! Damn! Damn!"

March 12

Ray lost bowel control again today. He was very upset and became depressed. I told him I loved him. I would love him always. He responded by saying, "I'm not worth loving. I'm nothing."

The other day as I was walking him down the stairs he said, "Take care of me, Honey. Take care of me."

March 16

Ray was up all night moaning, cursing, crying, and tossing. Once he said, "I feel like killing myself. Where will this end?" I could do nothing. But I know that if Ray could understand what is happening to him, and have the power, he would choose death. He got up a couple of times and wandered around aimlessly. He hasn't done that in a long time. And it scares me because he falls. I held him, but that did not comfort him, and only served to make it harder for me. How can you distance yourself, not feel pain, when you're holding on to and caring for the very thing you are losing?

The next morning David dressed Ray while I prepared breakfast. I was in the kitchen when I heard David helping Ray down the steps. Then I heard David say, "Oh, Daddy!" and the heavy thump of Ray falling. When I got to him, he was on his back, his stomach and right side jerking involuntarily. His face was expressionless. I didn't know what was wrong, but within a couple of minutes it passed, and we helped him down the stairs. I went on to work, tense and afraid. I knew I could lose him at any time. Late in the afternoon Ben called. He was concerned about how agitated Ray was. Ben had never called me at work before, which made me feel there was reason for concern.

When I got home Ray was upstairs lying down. Ben and I talked a few minutes. When he left, I phoned Dr. Thornton, a family practitioner Marjorie had recommended to me before she left.

As I gave the doctor a sketchy outline of Ray's history, Ray got up and came out into the hall. I could see, but I couldn't reach him. As I watched, he seemed to lose his balance; then I saw and heard his head strike the wall. I dropped the phone and rushed to his side. His face was contorted and twitching. He fell to the floor. I ran back to the phone and Jim, our tenant, who somehow appeared on the scene, went to Ray.

I was hysterical, but I described what was happening to the doctor. "He's having a grand mal seizure," he told me. He instructed me to call an ambulance and meet him at the hospital. I was of no use to Ray or Jim. Ray had completed his seizure and gone into a very deep sleep. I ran around the house, looking for copies of medical records I had. I knew the doctor knew nothing about Ray except for what I had briefly told him on the phone. Then I ran outside to see if the ambulance had arrived and back into the house, wondering if I should get out of my sweatsuit. I found out later that there is little anyone can do to help someone who has had a seizure; that's a relief, because I was a basket case. The ambulance arrived within minutes. Ray's blood pressure was high, but his vital signs were stable.

In the emergency room the doctors gave Ray Dilantin to control the seizures, did a CAT scan to check if he had suffered a subdural hematoma, and then admitted him to the hospital. He was to be monitored for a couple of days on the Dilantin, have an electroencephalogram to check for brain damage, and then be released. I didn't understand what the seizure meant and I was worried about Ray. At the same time I was looking forward to the few days Ray would be in the hospital. I would be able to get a full night's sleep, and leave the house when and for as long as I wanted to. I knew Ray would be cared for. It was as if I had a three-day pass.

I decided to visit Ray during mealtimes so that I could feed him. I knew that a visit without a purpose would not mean much to him. I felt somewhat guilty, but enjoyed the freedom. I knew, too, that I would have to deal with the problems that we would encounter when Ray came home. His falling so frequently made me realize that we needed to restructure how much and where he walked to avoid his seriously hurting himself. It was at this point, for the first time, that I decided that it was time to at least place Ray's name on nursing home waiting lists. I didn't know how much longer it was safe for him to be at home.

But Sunday morning, just a day and a half after Ray had been admitted, Dr. Thornton called. As he was speaking with me, he was reviewing some blood and urine test results that he had just received on Ray. In the middle of the conversation he stopped. His tone changed. He told me that the test results he was looking at showed that Ray was in kidney failure. He said that he'd get back to me after he conferred with a kidney specialist. I hung up the telephone. I knew what decision I would be asked to make.

I called two physicians: my brother-in-law and a neighbor. As objectively and as accurately as I could, I reported the happenings of the last two days and waited for their response. Both gave me the same advice. Do nothing. No dialysis. No emergency medical assistance. I knew that decision meant Ray would die. But the alternative would be crueler: dialysis for the rest of his life to maintain a life that by any standard had only minimal quality. I knew what Ray would do. I knew what I must do. But it was hard to be the one to actually say, "Do nothing. Let him go."

I spoke with the doctors on and off all that day. The message was that, without dialysis, Ray had one week to live.

I had known it would come. I had thought about it often, but did not think it would happen this way—so suddenly, so soon. Was I ready? Is there ever a time when we are really ready?

I was too scared to cry. There was so much to do. I had to stay strong. I had to know what was happening. I had to make the right decisions.

And so the end began. At first he was agitated and irritable; I spent most of my short visits in the hall in tears. I knew Ray did not know what he was saying, but that did not lessen the hurt. Over the next few days Ray ate less and less, until he ate or drank nothing at all. When the Dilantin was stopped, the seizures started. The doctors said it was a choice of deaths. If they continued the Dilantin, it would poison his system because he could not excrete it through his kidneys. Without the Dilantin he would continue to have seizures and would die of uremic poisoning because of the failure of his kidneys.

I soon was able to recognize the warning symptoms of a seizure. The nurses kept a supply of six or seven padded tongue depressors taped onto the wall for ready availability, and often I was the only one in the room. There was no place for paralysis and hysteria. And, although my throat tightened, my heart pounded, and my hands shook, I quickly learned how to place the tongue depressor in Ray's mouth so that he did not bite his tongue. But there were times when he seemed to take so long coming out of the seizure that I thought he wouldn't make it. I would stand there, sometimes a nurse or two with me. "Oh, God, no," I would cry, "not yet, please not yet. Not like this." I realized that we hang on to even the slenderest threads of life, unwilling to let any one of them go.

Gradually, Ray slipped into a deepening coma, a kind of anesthetized sleep. But it was not the peaceful coma state I had expected. Ray was wasting away on the outside, and inside he was dying of uremic poisoning. The seizures continued, and his breathing became what is called Cheyne-Stokes breathing: periods of deep abdominal breathing followed by periods of not breathing.

The boys came. I wanted them to see Ray just one more time. I felt that would help finalize it for them, as I hoped it would for me.

I found that now, as the end neared, I had to be there. I'm not sure why, but somehow it was important that I be with him during those final hours. I knew that every time I left the hospital, it could be the last time I would see Ray. But, if possible, I wanted to be there.

I felt no regrets for what was, no if-only's, no guilt (maybe a little in the earlier stages over the anger I had felt toward Ray when he had really been doing the best he could). Yes, Ray was too young. Yes, I would miss him desperately. But his life had been good. He had wonderful memories of his childhood. He was valued and fulfilled by his family. He had received many accolades in his profession. We had not put our life off until . . . whenever.

My parents came from Florida and were with me the last few days. On a rainy Saturday night, we left the hospital unsure if Ray would be alive the next morning. It was raining, and the parking lot was empty. As we walked to the car, my parents offered, as they had before, to stay longer if I wanted them to. They were anxious to help in any way they could. I said no, that we needed to get some rest. But I knew that Ray could go during the night and I wouldn't be there. By the time we got to the car, I could barely contain the suffering within me.

My mother assured me again that they would be glad to go back and wait. I could hold it in no longer. I started to scream hysterically, "It's no use! It doesn't matter anymore! He's going to die! He's going to die!" I drove home, crying uncontrollably for the few miles to our house, my father trying to calm me, my mother afraid to utter a word for fear she'd make it worse.

My poor parents didn't know what to do or say. I know they would have done anything within their power to help me, but couldn't. We came into the house and I went into the bedroom and cried. I'm not sure what I cried for. I imagine it was a bit of everything, but mostly I was crying for me—for my loss, my love, my life. I still couldn't believe it was happening, and yet I knew it was.

Somehow that release helped, and I went into my parents' room. I remember standing there and wanting them to hear, understand, and believe me. I knew they would go back to Florida and remember my pain, and hurt more than I wanted them to. And so, with tears still running down my cheeks I said, "I want you to know something." I said it strongly and clearly, with the kind of conviction I often had when I was trying to convince myself of something that I wasn't too sure of, but desperately wanted to believe. "I want you to know," I went on, "that no matter what you see in the next few days, be assured that I am going to be okay." I did believe that. I had to believe that. I don't think I could have thought about a life ahead enduring the agony I was in.

We got to the hospital about 7:30 the next morning. Ray's room was across the hall from the elevator. His door was open, and I cautiously walked toward the room. As I entered, I initially peeked in as I had done for the past few days. Then I inched in a step at a time, making sure Ray was still in the bed, that it was not over.

It was hard to tell if Ray was still there; he had lost so much weight that he hardly made a bulge under the sheet that covered him. As I entered that morning, I saw that his breathing was noticeably different. Breaths were short and each more like a single gasp, rather than part of a rhythmic breathing pattern. It seemed that he was getting little air to or from his lungs. His breathing was so labored that every breath seemed as if it might be his last. His eyes were red, and when they opened involuntarily, I could see them move from side to side, but not focus on anything. His face was jaundiced, and his skin had a crust on it that the doctor had said was from the uremic poisoning.

I could not move away from the side of his bed. I knew the end was near. I wanted to believe that somehow he had waited for me to be there with him. I could not utter a word to my parents. We were alone, Ray and I. He was probably unaware of my presence, but I couldn't leave. My knees shook and my heart pounded. I knew it wasn't going to be long. I was frightened, but I stroked his now bearded face and his hands, taking his last breaths with him. I told him again as I had so many times before how much I loved him. I thanked him for being part of my life and told him that I would never forget him.

I had never seen anyone die or even seen a corpse. I wanted to run, but I couldn't. I had to be there with him. I had always been there and would not leave him now.

As I stood watching, Ray seemed to take in less and less air until he was only sipping in air, as if through a straw. I was prepared to ring for the nurse when it was time. I would need someone there. I was frightened. I was watching my husband die. It wasn't a dream, a book, a movie. It was real. It would only be moments and the nightmare would be over.

In his final moments Ray seemed to have some facial seizuring; his face contorted and twitched; he was biting down on his tongue. I rang for the nurse. I held Ray's hand and begged him to let go. "Go my sweet. Be at peace. Know that you were loved. Let go."

The nurse entered, checked his eyes, and listened to his heart. His fingers were already blue. "He's gone, isn't he?" I asked.

"Not quite," she answered, and continued to watch and listen. In a few moments she turned to me and said, "He's gone."

It was over. He was at peace. No longer would he endure this disease which had so slowly, but relentlessly, destroyed him. No longer would we watch, helpless and hopeless. If death is ever a blessing, this was.

REFLECTIONS ONE YEAR LATER

I woke this morning and lay in bed with my eyes open for a few seconds before I realized that I had just had a dream. I dreamed that Ray had left me. He had just left. There was no discussion, no prior understanding, nothing. He had decided that he just didn't want to live with me anymore. He didn't say that he didn't love me. He didn't leave out of anger. But he was gone. I called him on the phone and begged him to come back. But he didn't answer. He didn't say anything. I called again. This time I told him that I hated him and that he was responsible for whatever happened to me because of what he had done. I had loved him and he had left me. He didn't even tell me why. I hadn't done anything. It wasn't fair. But what I couldn't do was stop loving him.

I lay in bed awhile assuring myself that it was a dream and that I could let go of the weight I felt on my chest. Ray didn't choose to leave. He didn't want to go. He didn't ask to go. It had just happened. Unknowingly he had slipped away. An insidious, destructive disease had invaded his body. It had ravaged his mind, destroying his very essence and leaving only a shell.

Ray and I never got to say good-bye. By the time we knew what was wrong, his ability to comprehend and express himself was so diminished that it was no longer possible. I had begged God to let him return to me so that we could exchange those last words—just for a few hours or even minutes. But it was too late.

Alone with Ray in the hospital during those last few moments, I told him what he meant to me and how I loved him, but I do not know that he heard. There had been many moments in the past when he did hear—when we shared our contentment and satisfaction with each other, when we joked

214

about what we would each do if the other died, knowing that the problem was years away and that we need not think seriously about it. Ray always knew how I felt, and he showed what I meant to him in many ways—an unexpected gift, a call in the middle of the day, his patience, tenderness, caring, and unconditional loving.

I would like to believe that as I stood beside him in those last moments, there was a deeper form of communication between us, something that transcended words. It consoles me to think that Ray was somehow aware of my presence, that he died knowing I was with him.

Elisabeth Kübler-Ross, a physician specializing in problems of dying patients and their families, has written that ideally there should be no unfinished business between ourselves and loved ones when we die or lose someone to death. She urges that nothing be left unsaid and nothing be left undone. With the exception of those words of farewell, there was nothing unsaid or undone between Ray and me. We had shared our love and frustration, our hopes and disappointments with each other.

But there remains unfinished business between myself and others. Perhaps this book is in part a means of finishing that business. I feel a compelling wish that those who misinterpreted the elusive and insidious signs, as I did, should understand that progressive brain deterioration often creates an erroneous picture of a victim. Consequently, changes in behavior and personality are misunderstood.

I ask others to learn as I have learned: to let Ray's life and death teach us. Let his futile struggle encourage us to search beyond superficial explanations.

It has been one year since Ray died. The autopsy report from Duke University Medical Center confirmed the diagnosis of Binswanger's disease. No definitive answers were reported about how Ray's heart or kidneys were involved in the disease process. But the knowledge gained from Ray about Binswanger's disease will further research; for that I am grateful.

I have been through one of each holiday, birthday, and anniversary, and have somehow endured. I have given Ray's clothes away, sorted through and discarded belongings I could let go of, and changed names on accounts (never, however, relinquishing Mrs. for Ms.). Slowly, Michael, David, and I are healing. Grieving is indeed the hard work that I was promised. But with time having passed, our memories now sometimes produce smiles rather than pain and tears.

I try not to dwell on "why us?" but instead on "what now?" In my journal I wrote many times of the living dead: those who give up and go through the motions of living, but really do no more than exist. I don't want, or intend, to be one of them. Still, I have periods when life does not seem important, when it is a struggle to find purpose and feel optimism. There is no one any longer to share joys and disappointments, no one with whom I can make a complete fool of myself, no one who lies next to me, no one who is totally there to share and listen. I have friends and family who love me, but I am alone. Maybe I am stronger, maybe even wiser, but I would not have traded Ray's life, and the peace, joy, and pleasure I found in our lives, for anything I have gained from this experience. Nonetheless, I am here. And now, oh God, what do I do with the rest of my life?

I fill up time beautifully: work, meetings, dinner with friends, trips, a dance class where I pretend to look like the graceful dancers pictured on the wall rather than the "astonishment" I see in the mirror before me. But the core of my life is gone.

Sometimes I feel that there is a hole in my existence, and I don't know how to fill it. I am afraid that the hole will remain empty and that the peripheral things that fill my life now will soon not prove to be enough. I allow myself to feel that these perceptions are temporary, that in time I will come to know fulfillment and serenity again.

Michael and David give me purpose. As they grow and mature, as they seek to find their own directions in life, I need to be a model for them. I don't try to hide my grief, but I also want them to see my resolve. I want them to know that their mother, like other women, is strong and resourceful.

Michael is a junior in college. He and I will attend David's high school graduation in a few days. I am profoundly sorry that Ray cannot be there. He will miss David in his white cap and gown walking to the stage to receive his diploma.

For David's graduation gift, I have framed a drawing Ray sent me many years ago: a detailed, sequential, ten-step "lesson" titled "How to draw a Nebbish." At the bottom of the page, Ray wrote, "Put them all together, they spell Nebbish—a man who is going nowhere—not quite a leader of men—yet still manages to run with the human race in his galoshes. He loves you. I love you."

I know I lost Ray long before he actually died. I lost the part of him that made him the man I found so satisfying. I did not fall in love with Ray because he was gorgeous—in today's slang, a "hunk." He wasn't. I'm not sure exactly what it was that drew us together. But I do know that we found completeness in each other. We complemented and balanced each other. As he deteriorated, we lost that. But there was a bond that went beyond what we understood. His outbursts of frustration and anger, his accusations, were sometimes painful to endure. But somewhere inside him, there remained a sense of trust. He became a child, then almost an infant, needing protection from a world in which he could no longer function. But he never ceased to belong to us.

Almost until the end, though, there remained those moments in which Ray's sense of humor, his painful and profound momentary awareness, and his fragments of preserved memory came together. In those precious, penetrating, infrequent moments, he could reach across the chasm and touch us. They were the remnants of what was, fragile threads that became precious treasures.

Through the writing of this book I have rethought and relived the progression of this story endless times, seeking answers, and understanding. I have been asked, and often I have asked myself, if it would have been better if we had known what was wrong with Ray earlier. I used to think that it would have been. But now I wonder. That is not to say that I would not have

217

wanted to know if the doctors knew. But perhaps not knowing enabled Ray and me to hang on longer—to preserve as long as possible what we had left in our lives together.

Surprisingly perhaps, I harbor little ill-feeling toward the well-intentioned professionals who misinterpreted the elusive signs and symptoms of Ray's disease and, consequently, could not accurately diagnose Ray's case. They operated within the limitations of their own disciplines and for the most part were not able to reach beyond those boundaries to seek alternative answers. Certainly such a difficult-to-diagnose disease would warrant the forming of a multi-disciplinary team, composed of a broad spectrum of professionals. Together they might have been able to identify the insidious, progressive nature of an organic brain disease, eliminate a psychological cause, and make an accurate diagnosis earlier.

Instead, much of the intervention that was attempted—five weeks in a psychiatric ward, marriage counseling, vitamin therapy, insertion of a shunt—was as useless as it was well intentioned; in fact, it created complications, added emotional trauma, and subjected Ray to unneeded physical risk.

For example, Ray spent almost five weeks in a psychiatric ward. He did not seem to find it a bad experience. But the stay seems to me to have been unusually long. I still don't understand why a CAT scan wasn't done right away, rather than after four weeks. We might have avoided some of the confusion and turmoil of that period.

"Marriage therapy" only added more problems and misunderstandings. I am not sure I will ever forgive myself for driving away from the hospital the day I came to pick Ray up for a haircut. He had forgotten to come down and meet me, so I left, believing that it was for the best. Dr. Hudson had told us that Ray really was strong—that he was very controlling while seeming to be dependent. I could be most helpful by making him responsible for himself and less reliant on me. But in my heart I knew that driving away that day was wrong. That was one time I truly abandoned him, and I am still very sorry I did. When we are in great need, we can become vulnerable to others' perceptions—even when we are right and they are wrong.

I found the idea of vitamin therapy as a treatment for dementia a strange one. Listening to the doctor's encouraging prognosis brightened our outlook, but the diagnosis was made on poor evidence and perhaps even wishful thinking. The months after Ray's first hospital stay were probably the most difficult of all because of that diagnosis and the false hope it offered.

I was torn between feeling that Ray was somehow in complicity with what was happening and a gnawing sense that his lack of "fight" was beyond his control. Dr. Townsend said Ray just needed to lead a healthier life. I would rather have faced the truth at that point. It would have devastated us, but it was more painful to live with the stress of believing that Ray would get well soon. I made it harder for Ray during that time—I expected more than he was capable of. His words—"I can't give you what you want"—still ring in my ears.

The operation to insert a shunt also was a useless intervention. I should probably have sought a second opinion. But at least I was aware of the slim odds that Ray would improve.

I have been asked if in looking back I feel foolish or guilty for initially attempting to hold Ray responsible for what was happening. I regret that, because I did not understand what was wrong earlier, I must have made things harder for him. I thought, or at least wanted to think, that he could control what was happening. But I didn't know. There were times when Ray would tell me that what was wrong was physical—such as the day he said he wanted to tell the auto mechanic that he was brain-damaged. I dismissed those observations—why I'm not sure. But clearly at that point there was little objective evidence. I could not conceive of Ray's losing his greatest gift, his mind.

I don't feel guilty—at least I have now forgiven myself. I do wish I hadn't told Ray that Michael had taken over the mowing because he acted so helpless. I wish I hadn't signed us up for the computer course that was so upsetting to Ray. But it's the nature of organic brain disease—Binswanger's, Alzheimer's, or any of the other causes of progressive, irreversible brain deterioration—that the onset is more clearly (and frequently only) seen in retrospect.

As long as I felt that Ray was somehow responsible (and I held on to that even after I knew that his illness was organically based) I could feel hope—some power to regain a life that I saw slipping away faster than I could comprehend. It was only gradually, as I was forced to face Ray's total inability to control what was happening, that I began to shift my thinking to my own survival.

I think the turning point was the day Ray and I worked on the computer at the public library. I was struck by his utter confusion and frustration as he tried to do something beyond his ability. I knew then that he was not in control of what was happening. My anger and my expectations began to subside. But as I let go of the anger, and stopped fighting to bring Ray back, did I also let go of part of his humanity? Were my anger and expectations, though they could not affect Ray, somehow mechanisms by which I could endure?

My dreams are beginning to change. Before, they always included Ray. He was their focus, their direction. Now they have no limits, no boundaries. Unidentified people appear; often I envision myself with someone—a man. He stands next to me, but he has no features, no physical description, no identifiable personality traits. Sometimes I fantasize that someone will appear in my waking life, swooping me away to a life of happiness forever after. But I can't spend a lifetime waiting for another knock on the door.

To a large extent, we are responsible for our own happiness. There is no Prince Charming, no fairy godmother, no magic lamp. There is only me, and I must gather whatever resources I have and begin to carve out a new beginning. I must use what I learned from Ray, and what I have learned about myself from the long ordeal of his dying, to forge ahead, in a direction yet unknown. Although it is frightening to stand at the door of a new life, a part of me anxiously awaits what it may possibly offer. Slowly, I am opening the door.

APPENDIX

The Medical History of Ray Doernberg
(b. 8 March 1936–d. 25 March 1984)

1945
—Diagnosis of rheumatic fever; develops functional heart murmur
—Following recovery, experiences pain in feet, knees, and shoulder; chronic pain in shoulders persists into adulthood; pain controlled with aspirin until mid-1970s

Mid-1970s
—Begins taking stronger analgesics, including Percodan and Darvocet N; continues to do so until about March 1982

April 1977
—Experiences inability to speak for a period of about ten minutes

1979-1982
—Seeks psychological help

October 1981
—Experiences numbness on right side of body
—CAT scan and waking EEG do not reveal abnormalities
—Persantine prescribed

18 March 1982
—Experiences swelling in feet and ankles

19 May 1982
—Kidney biopsy performed
—Analgesic nephritis diagnosed
—No treatment prescribed; advised not to use analgesics

9 September 1982
—Undergoes psychological testing
—Results of IQ testing: verbal 113, performance 79, full-scale 96

9 September-14 October 1982
—Placed in psychiatric ward; no psychiatric findings
—CAT scan reveals fluid in brain
—Vitamin therapy recommended as treatment

6 January 1983
—Second battery of tests including psychological tests and CAT scan
—Results of IQ testing: verbal 109, performance 74, full-scale 92
—Normal pressure hydrocephalus diagnosed

31 January-12 February 1983
—Cardiac catheterization performed to determine if pacemaker would be necessary before implantation of shunt; no cardiac intervention indicated
—Ventriculo-peritoneal shunt implanted

12 May 1983
— Third set of psychological tests administered
—Results of IQ testing: verbal 84, performance 57, full-scale 71

10 July-23 July 1983
—Admitted to Duke University Medical Center
—Third-degree heartblock necessitates implantation of pacemaker
—Diagnosis of Binswanger's disease (subcortical arteriosclerotic encephalopathy)

17 March 1984
—Hospitalized after grand mal seizure at home
—Tests reveal kidney failure; no dialysis

25 March 1984
—Dies of kidney failure
—Autopsy report confirms diagnosis of Binswanger's disease